To my girls, Rowen and Greer, you have been my greatest gift.

HOW TO HAVE
HOPE
WHEN THERE IS
NO CURE

A Comprehensive Guide
to Chronic Pain Rehabilitation

Murray J. McAllister, PsyD

How to Have Hope When There Is No Cure: A Comprehensive
Guide to Chronic Pain Rehabilitation

Copyright © 2023 by Murray J. McAllister, PsyD

Printed in the United States of America
Hardcover ISBN: 979-8-218-22505-6
Paperback ISBN: 979-8-218-22506-3
Ebook ISBN: 979-8-218-22507-0

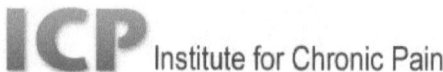 Institute for Chronic Pain

The Institute for Chronic Pain is an educational and public policy think tank whose
mission is to make pain management more effective by changing the culture of how
chronic pain is treated. We engage in research, development, and promotion of
scientifically accurate information related to the field of chronic pain management.
We do so by bringing together thought leaders from around the world to provide
academic-quality information that is approachable to all stakeholders in the field.

https://www.instituteforchronicpain.org

Table of Contents

What Is the Goal and How Do We Get There?

Believe it or not, people have chronic pain and aren't upset by it. They aren't angry, anxious, or depressed about it. They don't typically avoid doing things that hurt. Instead, they know what their pain is and what to do about it. They stay on top of it because they know how to deal with pain really well. In fact, they deal with it so well that pain just occurs in the background as they go about their daily activities.

Now, of course, they may have made lifestyle changes to deal with pain well, but they aren't upset by these changes. They may no longer ski in the winter. They may have stopped long-distance running or playing softball in a local community league. They may have even changed positions at work to better accommodate for the pain. Nonetheless, they still go to work every day. They still do fun things with friends and family. They sleep at night. They do chores at home. Their relationships with their spouse and kids are good.

They might also do things that they never used to do. They walk for exercise on a regular basis. They do some type of daily relaxation exercise. They make it a point to manage their stress well. They pace their daily activities. They may have made a number of these kinds of lifestyle changes since their pain became chronic.

Again, though, they aren't upset about these changes. In fact, they may have even come to a point where they like doing these things. It makes life easier. It helps to manage pain. They know it too and, as a result, it maintains their motivation to do these things almost every day.

All of this is to say that some people manage chronic pain really well, even though they have made quite a few changes in their lives to deal with it. When asked about who they are or how they are doing, they talk about their family, job, or activities. It might not even occur to them to mention that they have chronic pain.

What would it be like to put chronic pain into the background of your life like that?

How do they do it? Some people just naturally do it. Other people have to learn. There's no shame in needing to learn. Some people naturally bowl or play basketball better than others and we never give it much thought if we're some of those people who aren't naturally athletic. Likewise, if you're someone who doesn't naturally deal with chronic pain well, don't be ashamed or embarrassed. You aren't doing anything wrong. Really! At this point, don't give it too much thought. Later, we'll talk more about how different people deal with pain and the stigma that can come along with it in our society.

The point here is that it's possible. People can learn to manage chronic pain so well that it is no longer upsetting to live with chronic pain. They have chronic pain and yet they're involved and engaged in their lives. They work full-time. They have relationships that are meaningful and satisfying. In other words, they are engaged in their lives and have no more or no less stress and problems than anyone else has.

This description is our goal.

You too can learn to do it. In healthcare, we call it *self-management*. In general, self-management is a two-pronged approach to managing any kind of chronic health problem, whether it's pain, heart disease, diabetes, or any other chronic condition. The two prongs are healthy lifestyle changes and increasing your ability to cope with the condition. By doing these things and practicing them over time, you get so good at dealing with the condition that it's no longer a major problem in your life.

Now, when it comes to chronic pain conditions, specifically, where you learn the two-pronged approach to self-management is in *chronic pain rehabilitation programs*. In such programs, you learn that the two prongs are a) a number of lifestyle changes that, when done over time, reduce pain by positively affecting its physiological bases and b) increasing your abilities to internally cope with the pain that will remain. The purposes of these two strategies are to reduce pain and to reduce its impact on you. In other words, you'll still have pain, but it will no longer be a major problem in your life.

This book aims to tell you how to do it. It also aims to make chronic pain rehabilitation familiar so that you and your family can know that help is available. Taking back your life and self-managing pain is possible. People learn how to do it every day in chronic pain rehabilitation programs.

Chronic pain rehabilitation programs

So what are chronic pain rehabilitation programs (CPRPs)? They're a traditional form of chronic pain management that focus on self-management. They're intensive. They provide multiple therapies on a daily basis over three or four weeks. They are interdisciplinary, meaning that the staff consists of psychologists, physicians, physical therapists, and nurses. Sometimes, they may also have occupational therapists, social workers, and vocational rehabilitation specialists.

They typically have nine core therapies to them. These core components are the following:

- Daily pool therapy
- Daily stretching and core strengthening
- Daily mild, low-impact aerobic exercise
- Daily relaxation therapies
- Daily coping skills training
- Weekly individual psychotherapy
- Individualized non-narcotic medication management (particularly the use of antidepressants and antiepileptics)
- Individualized tapering of narcotic medications as needed
- Life/work exposure therapy

Unless indicated, these therapies are done in small groups of patients. In the following chapters, we'll discuss these core components, not only how to do them, but how they are helpful.

Common reactions to hearing about chronic pain rehabilitation programs

When first hearing about CPRPs, some patients respond that they've already tried the core therapies. They might say, for instance, that they've tried physical therapy soon after initially getting injured and they may have tried it a few times since then too. They might also say that they've seen a psychologist or that they've tried a number of different non-narcotic medications, but pain and disability remained. They also frequently say that they tried to stop taking narcotic pain medications in the past, but their pain became too intense and so resumed taking them. The upshot of all these responses is something like the following: what's so special about doing these therapies in a CPRP?

To answer, we might recall the old saying about the whole being greater than the sum of its parts. Sometimes, of course, the old saying is true and it's certainly true when it comes to CPRPs. Patients typically have done most of these therapies, but they've done them on an individual basis, at different times in the history of their pain, and often without coordination between providers. What goes on in a CPRP has two important differences:

- The therapies are coordinated by an interdisciplinary team of healthcare providers
- All nine therapies are done on a daily basis across three to four weeks, which simulates real life

Doing the therapies in this manner makes all the difference.

First, you learn everything you need to know in a coordinated fashion. It's like going to chronic pain school. The interdisciplinary staff is like the different teachers of a school, teaching you how to live well despite having chronic pain. The fact that all therapies are done on the same day, every day, across three to four weeks gives you the opportunity to learn the two prongs of self-management and practice them well before going off on your own.

Second, it does more than that and here's the crucial part. The fact that all the therapies are done on the same day, every day, across three to four weeks, teaches patients how to be active for up to a full day, every day. It's a way to practice returning to an active life on a daily basis. Like no other pain treatment, CPRPs show people how to get back into life and/or return to work, because you're essentially doing it in the program. That is to say, CPRPs simulate getting back into real life, work included. You're taught how to do it by a team of experts who coach and support you along the way. After a number of weeks, patients learn how to maintain the daily activities of life. They also regain the confidence that they really can do it. That's the crucial difference. It's what makes the whole greater than the sum of its parts.

What I just described is the ninth core component of CPRPs – life/work exposure therapy. Even if you've done the other core therapies, you haven't done this last one, unless you've participated in a CPRP. Doing the other therapies on an individual basis at different times in the history of your care is often insufficient to learn how to get back into life while self-managing your pain. One hour, weekly physical therapy or pain psychology appointments just isn't similar enough to your real life or your full-time job to learn how to return to them on a full-time basis– all the while keeping your pain under control.

The life/work exposure therapy within a CPRP makes the crucial difference because CPRPs are similar enough to real life. When you attend a program, you put yourself in a position to allow a team of experts to teach you how to be active for up to a full day for a number of weeks on end while at the same time managing your pain well. Most patients won't ever learn to do it until they participate in a CPRP. Moreover, you not only learn how to do it; you regain the confidence that you really can do it. Learning in a supportive environment with a team of experts, you come to see that you really can take back your life.

I often tell patients that participating in a CPRP is going to be one of the most empowering experiences they'll ever have.

However, when I recommend and describe CPRPs to patients for the first time, they often react with protests that they'd never be able to do it. They're too disabled, they say, to do anything for a full day, let alone every day for a number of weeks. You might be saying it right now as you read this introduction. Nevertheless, I'd ask you to consider the following description of a typical patient who succeeds in a CPRP:

- A person who has at least one chronic pain condition lasting for years, and has been unable to work for some time
- A person who struggles to do daily chores and may have difficulty even doing the basics of life, like standing or walking for too long
- A person who, in addition to having chronic pain, experiences insomnia, irritability, anxiety, depression, and/or strained relationships

As you can tell, CPRPs are set up to help the most disabled and distressed people with chronic pain. And they succeed in doing it. Indeed, CPRPs are considered one of the most effective treatments for those with chronic pain (Gatchel & Okifuji, 2006; Turk, 2002).

If the above typical patient describes you, at least in part, then you can succeed in taking back your life too. You just have to give it a chance and learn how.

Are you ready?

How this book should be used

Let's look at how this book is set up and how it can be used because it can be used in a number of ways.

First, it can be used as a companion guide to your participation in a CPRP. While in these programs, it's often helpful for patients to read about how chronic pain can be treated. As you progress through the program, your treatment providers can assign chapters to read as a way to reinforce what you learn in your therapies. Or the chapters might introduce new ideas, which you can later discuss with your providers.

The sections and chapters are written in a progressive manner to be read from start to finish, building on each other and roughly following the progression of a typical CPRP. However, they're also written as short sections, which can stand on their own and be easily read individually as assignments. Your treatment providers might jump around from section to section, based on your progress or your individualized needs.

Second, this book is also a guide for your CPRP provider. It's what's called a *treatment manual* for CPRPs. No treatment manual is widely available to guide these programs and provide a standardized protocol and rationale for them.

Third, we know that CPRPs aren't available in all areas of the world and at times health insurance may not cover them. The sad truth is that, while CPRPs are one of the most effective forms of pain management, many patients don't have access to them because of either a lack of programs in their area or adequate insurance coverage. As such, some patients end up pursuing pain rehabilitation on an individual basis with different providers at the same time. In such situations, it'll be helpful to read this book as a stand-alone self-help book.

As such, this book is written to be an intervention all by itself – to motivate you to make changes in your life so that you can deal with chronic pain more effectively. The emphasis here is on what you can do to get better. As such, there's nothing in the following pages for which you absolutely need to be in a clinic to learn. For the motivated chronic pain sufferer, this book can be your guide to taking back control of your life.

Who might benefit from this book?

The answer is the same whether you're using this book as a guide to participating in a formal CPRP or using it as a stand-alone self-help book. It's for people with chronic pain. As we'll see, it's often hard for people to accept that their pain is chronic, but let's try to clarify how the phrase *chronic pain* is used in this book.

Chronic pain isn't just any pain, but rather pain that meets two rough criteria. First, this book is for people whose pain has lasted more than six months. The time frame of six months is a rule of thumb in common use among healthcare providers who specialize in pain management because most acute injuries or illnesses will have healed by then. The second criterion for what chronic pain means in this book is that the pain is due to health conditions that are not terminal. Common examples are low back pain, neck pain, recurrent headaches or migraines, fibromyalgia, arthritis, neuropathy, or complex regional pain syndrome. Notice that none of these conditions lead to death, which is what *terminal* means. So, chronic pain refers in this book to the pain of health conditions which you may have for the rest of your life, and when in fact it does come time to pass away, you'll die with them and not from them.

There is one more point to make about who'll benefit from this book. Briefly put, it's that you have to be interested in what you can do to get better. As we'll see, there's a time and place for relying on healthcare providers to make you better, but there's also a time and place for you, the chronic pain patient, to learn what you can do to reduce pain and its impact on you. As a patient, if you see your role as solely finding the right specialist to make you well, then this book is not for you. But, if you're willing to entertain the idea that it would be helpful to learn what *you can do* to get better, even if it doesn't cure you, then this book is for you.

The goal of chronic pain rehabilitation programs

So, what is our goal? The aim of this book is to help you to deal with chronic pain so successfully that despite having chronic pain you are no more stressed or disabled than anyone else is – even people without chronic pain. In other words, our goal is for you to be involved and engaged in your life, work, and relationships, and find them to be meaningful and satisfying – at least to the extent that they are for anyone else in life – even those without chronic pain.

Notice that it isn't a super lofty goal. No one is promising divine bliss here. Nor are you promised a pain-free life. Our goal is just to get somewhere into the normal range of functioning in life despite having chronic pain.

The normal range of life is still hard at times. Good things happen. Bad things happen. People get stressed and depressed or anxious. People stop doing things that they once enjoyed and find new things to do. Life comes with these problems. Our goal in a CPRP is not to get away from these normal problems of life. Rather, our goal is to get to a point where you're not overly stressed or disabled by chronic pain. It's possible to have chronic pain that isn't overwhelming or disabling, but you have to learn how. By learning to effectively deal with it, you get to the point where the good and bad things that normally happen in life are what occupy your time and energy – not chronic pain.

While it's not a super lofty goal, it is difficult to achieve. It's going to take hard work on your part. It's also going to take time. There are no easy and quick fixes for chronic pain. But, you know that. If your pain had been quickly or easily fixed, you wouldn't be reading this book or seeking the help of a CPRP. Motivation and perseverance in making personal changes over time are the strongest predictors of who is successful in chronic pain rehabilitation.

So, again, are you ready?

CHAPTER ONE

The Place of Chronic Pain Rehabilitation in the Healthcare System

Sometimes, patients don't understand how chronic pain rehabilitation will help them. Perhaps it's when they meet with a rehabilitation provider for an initial evaluation or perhaps it's in the first few days of attending a CPRP, but this lack of understanding tends to keep them from fully participating. They might, for instance, forgo recommendations or not give it their all. They do so because pain rehabilitation just doesn't make sense to them.

It's not uncommon for people to understand healthcare as something you rely on to get well. They see the role of the healthcare provider as someone who does therapies or procedures to you in order to get you better. In other words, it's common to think that what's going to get you better in the healthcare system are procedures and pills and the providers who deliver them.

When thinking about healthcare in this way, CPRPs don't seem to make a lot of sense. Where are the procedures and pills that are going to make you well? The healthcare providers in CPRPs don't seem to do anything to their patients in order to make them better.

Notice the subtle emphasis on what makes patients well. If you think that the sole role of healthcare is to do things to you in order to make you better, then it's hard to understand how a CPRP is going to help. As such, we need to clarify how CPRPs work. We need to show how there's another way to get better than simply relying on the healthcare system to do it for you. In short, we need to show how to change the focus of your care away from what the healthcare system can do for you and toward what you can do for yourself. Indeed, if you can see that you have an important role in getting better, then CPRPs are going to make a lot more sense. After all, CPRPs are where people go to learn what they can do to get better.

In this chapter, we'll focus on how the healthcare system has long been set up to provide two kinds of care: care that we rely on to get us well and care that we rely on to teach us how to get better ourselves. It's important to understand the place that CPRPs have in the greater healthcare system because it allows you to have confidence in its methods. You'll understand that CPRPs are not some new, unproven, alternative therapy, but rather have a long-held tradition of care with many years of scientific research proving their effectiveness. In doing so, we begin the necessary process of changing the emphasis of care from what the healthcare system can do for you to what you can do for yourself. In the next chapter, we'll continue this process by specifically focusing on what you can do to change your internal perspectives on how to get better. Our initial goals for these first two chapters are to take ownership of your health and well-being and thereby set the stage for committing to lifestyle changes that when done over time will reduce your pain and its impact on you.

The healthcare system at a glance

When it comes to treatments and therapies for health problems, our healthcare system has two broadly defined approaches. One is the acute medical model. Patients pursue this approach most often when seeking healthcare services. I like to call it *the fix-it model*. The second is the rehabilitation or *self-management* model. Patients pursue this approach less often, even though they could benefit from it more than the acute medical model, at least for some health conditions. It may be due to the fact that it's typically not as well understood by patients. Let's review both, one at a time.

Acute medical model, or the fix-it model

The acute medical model of healthcare is what we tend to think of as standard healthcare and in large measure we are right. When we get sick or injured, we go to a healthcare provider and a few different things occur, which we have all come to expect. First, we describe to the provider our symptoms and how we became injured or ill. We then undergo a physical examination. Following this history and physical, the provider performs a procedure or prescribes medicine, which acts upon us. The goal of submitting to the examination and undergoing these procedures or taking medicine is to get cured of what ails us. That is to say, we are presently sick or injured and we want to get back to how we were before we became ill or injured.

Now, when this type of healthcare works, it is a wonderful thing. With advances in science and technology, many ailments have come to be curable. Antibiotics cure bacterial infections. A cast can return a broken arm to normal. A surgery can cure potentially life-threatening appendicitis. Certain types of cancer are now curable with combinations of surgery, radiation, and chemotherapies. The fix-it model is truly a wonderful thing and it is testimony to its achievements that it has become the standard model of care: when we think of healthcare, we tend to think of the acute medical model.

Sometimes, of course, a cure isn't immediately available and a provider delivering care within the acute medical model will provide *symptom relief.* This approach is a little different than trying to fix the patient's illness or injury, but it is a healthcare approach that nonetheless lies within the acute medical model. When a fix to a patient's problem isn't immediately obvious, a provider will begin to try various things to fix the problem and this process will essentially be one of trial and error. The provider will try one thing after another until hitting upon the procedure or medication that fixes the problem. During this process, the provider might prescribe a medication, say, that won't exactly cure the patient but will in the meantime help the patient to feel better. Such symptom management is intended to be temporary until the cure is found. For example, we might take medication to reduce the symptom of a fever while also taking an antibiotic to cure underlying pneumonia. The fever-reducing medication is intended to be for symptom relief and the antibiotic is intended as a cure.

By the way, this is often the initial intention behind prescribing narcotic pain medications for chronic pain. A primary care provider might pursue pain symptom relief with narcotic medications while he or she sends you to different types of specialists – neurologists, interventional pain physicians, surgeons, or physical therapists – who will attempt to cure your pain. Sometimes, such specialists will take over prescribing the medications, but whoever prescribes them, the medications are intended to provide temporary pain symptom management until a cure can be found.

Other times, of course, there is no cure for what ails us and all healthcare providers do is symptom management. Many acute medical problems are managed in this way. The healthcare provider prescribes some type of treatment that is designed to keep a patient comfortable while the body naturally heals. Consider, for instance, when we experience a cold. We might take prescribed or over-the-counter medications to reduce the cough and congestion that we experience from a cold virus. Over a period of time, our bodies fight off the virus and we naturally return to how we were before we caught the cold.

In these cases of symptom management, the acute medical model provides needed care even when there is no actual fix for the medical problem that we might have. All of us, it could easily be assumed, are grateful for such symptom management therapies.

The strengths of the acute medical model are that for many types of ailments, it can provide a cure. When there are no cures, it can provide measures that help us feel better. In our society, we have come to equate healthcare with the acute medical model because of its significant strengths and successes, which we have all experienced.

The rehabilitation model

Despite these strengths, there are some types of illnesses and injuries that do not lend themselves well to a fix-it model approach. What are they? They are some of the most significant health problems of our day: heart disease, diabetes, and chronic pain. While each of these disorders is actually quite different from one another, they all have something in common. They are chronic health conditions.

A chronic health condition is one in which there is no cure and so it continues indefinitely. While medical procedures are sometimes pursued with these conditions, the most important thing in the management of chronic conditions is what patients do in terms of their health behaviors.

We might be most familiar with this emphasis on the patient's self-care in relation to heart disease or diabetes. In heart disease, a patient might have a heart attack and subsequently pursue a number of symptom-relieving strategies, such as a cardiac surgical procedure and high blood pressure and high cholesterol medications. However, we all know that if the patient doesn't also pursue certain lifestyle changes, these medical procedures and therapies will likely be ineffective to one degree or another. In heart disease, these changes that the patient must pursue are acceptance of the chronicity of the disorder, weight loss, changes in diet, exercise, smoking cessation, and stress management, among others. Similarly, in the case of diabetes, a patient might take medications, but again these medications will be largely ineffective if the patient doesn't also make certain lifestyle changes, such as acceptance of the chronicity of the disorder, changes in diet, weight loss, exercise, and stress management.

Chronic pain is similar. Most chronic pain patients have pursued symptom relief through numerous medical procedures but these are largely ineffective in relation to what patients themselves can do to manage chronic pain. These ways to self-manage pain are acceptance of the chronicity of the pain; regular aerobic exercise; stretching and strengthening exercises; regular relaxation exercises; increasing one's own coping strategies; reducing any related anxiety, depression, or insomnia; stress management; tapering narcotic pain medications; and returning to some type of productive activity.

At this point, we could expand on what these conditions have in common. Besides the fact that they are chronic, successful management of these conditions depends in large measure on what the patient does to get better and not so much on what healthcare providers do to get the patient better. This point lies at the heart of the rehabilitation model of care. The chief ways by which the rehabilitation model is helpful is by helping you to make lifestyle changes to best manage the chronic health condition you have. The emphasis is not on what healthcare providers can do for you, but on what you can do for you. Because of this emphasis on making changes in your life, the rehabilitation model is often also called the *self-management* model.

Because chronic conditions are, well, chronic, the goal of self-management is not to fix them, but to reduce the impact that the conditions have on you. Healthcare providers use a phrase to describe this goal: it is to reduce the *distress and impairment* that the condition causes. Distress and impairment is a phrase that refers to the adverse emotional and functional impact that a condition has on you, whether the impact is emotional, psychological, physical, occupational, financial, or social. Without using the phrase, we talked about reducing distress and impairment when describing our goal in the introduction of this book. We said that our goal is to get to the point where you are no longer upset about living with chronic pain and that you are able to get back engaged in your life, work, and relationships. The successful management of a chronic health condition is to accept its chronicity and adjust to it so well that you reduce its emotional and physical impact on you. In other words, metaphorically, you relegate pain from being your co-star to one of the extras in the movie that you call your life.

The goal of pain rehabilitation, then, is not to cure, but rather to foster acceptance of pain and educate patients to reduce its impact on them. The words of a patient best capture the goal of the rehabilitation model: "I've really come to accept it and have been able to move on with my life. Yes… my life has changed, but my chronic pain no longer runs my life. I do."

At this point, we can describe other differences between the fix-it model of care and the rehabilitation model. The ideal of the acute medical model is the quick fix. The fix produces a qualitative difference in the patient: you go from a state of illness or injury to a state of health. Getting better means returning to how you were the day before you became ill or injured. None of this is true in the rehabilitation model. There are no quick fixes here. It is a long, slow process of getting better over time. The ideal change is not qualitative but incremental. Getting better, therefore, means having less pain, less emotional distress about pain, better ability to sleep at night, being able to do more things, less need for narcotic pain medications, and so forth. The goal is not to return to how you were the day before it all started, but to get better from here, from where you are today, however you are, and to get better incrementally over time.

To reach such goals, many patients need help from healthcare providers: psychologists, physicians, physical therapists, and nurses, all of whom are rehabilitation specialists. We act not so much as a traditional doctor attempting to cure you, but as coaches who train you to move beyond the challenges of chronic pain. Within a friendly and trusting relationship, like you may have had with a coach, we train, teach, encourage, challenge, empower, and instill confidence that you can deal with your chronic pain and get beyond it by reducing its impact on you.

Again, notice that the emphasis is less on us and more on you. In the fix-it model of care, the patient is a passive recipient of the care that is provided. In the rehabilitation model, the patient is an active participant in the care. So, if we are your coaches, you are the athlete. Like any other athlete, to win the game – to get better – you have to perform. We coach, but you've got the ball. We will be with you to work through the defeats and challenges and also to celebrate the accomplishments, but you have the ball and are the one who has to run with it.

In our healthcare system, the traditional form of rehabilitation for chronic pain conditions occurs in CPRPs. For many years, CPRPs have been the traditional alternative to surgery or long-term narcotic pain medication management. Research has shown time and again that CPRPs are effective in helping people acquire the ability to successfully self-manage pain (Gatchel & Okifuji, 2006; Turk, 2002).

In the next chapter, we will go into more detail about the many underlying yet important concepts that make up the rehabilitation approach to chronic pain. It will be helpful to have a common vocabulary to use to continue our discussion into the subsequent chapters. In these chapters, we will review the many strategies and skill sets that you can learn to a) reduce pain by positively changing the physiological bases of your pain over time and b) increase your internal abilities to cope with the pain that may remain.

A final summary thought

Consider this thought the next time you have a quiet, reflective moment: if something in your life is a problem and over time you get so good at dealing with the problem that it no longer adversely affects you, then it remains in your life but it is no longer a problem. That is how you can get better even if pain remains chronic.

Believe it or not, people can get to the point where, over time and with hard work, they have accepted their pain and reduced its impact on their life and, as a result, living with chronic pain is no longer a problem for them.

Now, do they deal with it? – Certainly! Would they have chosen it? – Never! But are they distressed by it or consider themselves disabled by it? – Nope. In this sense, chronic pain comes to be no longer a problem. And if it is no longer a problem, then you no longer need to search in vain for a fix and you can move on with the rest of your life.

CHAPTER TWO

Taking Responsibility for
Your Health and Well-Being

By understanding the place that CPRPs have in the healthcare system, we come to see how chronic pain rehabilitation might be helpful even if it doesn't provide a cure. CPRPs have an established model of care that focuses on teaching you what to do in order to get better, incrementally over time. This focus entails that you take ownership of your health and well-being. You stop relying solely on healthcare providers to make you better and begin learning what you can do to get better yourself.

This shift is a change in perspective that leads to a change in what you do to get better. In other words, it's a cognitive and behavioral shift in how you manage chronic pain. In this way, we can see clearly how chronic pain rehabilitation is a two-pronged approach: it's a cognitive intervention whereby you learn to cope better with pain and it's a behavioral intervention whereby you learn lifestyle changes that over time reduce pain.

By shifting the focus from what healthcare providers can do for you to what you can do for yourself, you've already begun to change how you cope with pain. You're coming to see that you have an alternative to feeling helpless in response to pain and being dependent on healthcare providers to manage pain for you through acute medical care. In this chapter, let's continue the process of learning to cope better with pain. We'll do so by clarifying what coping is, what chronic pain is, how to accept it, and how to take ownership of its management. These concepts are essential to coping better with pain.

Coping better is a change in perspective

In healthcare, we consider learning to better cope with pain as a psychotherapeutic process. In everyday language, we just say that learning to cope better is about changing the perspective from which you see your problems. You change your understanding of them, which puts them in a new light, a light that allows you to see what to do about your problems. It's essentially a learning process.

To demonstrate how helpful it is to simply begin to see things differently, it might be best to take some everyday examples to illustrate the point. When I was a kid, we had a family friend from England who was a teacher here in America. When he had a break in the school year, and didn't have enough time to fly back home, he'd come to stay with us. He loved sports and, when he first arrived in America, baseball and American football were difficult for him to watch. He didn't understand them. He had a hard time knowing where the ball was or who had it. In his confusion, he'd sometimes become irritated, stop watching, and leave the room. I'd wonder if such experiences would lead him to miss his home in England and the past which he'd fondly remember: drinking a pint in the pub while cheering his favorite football (i.e. soccer) team. However, once he began to learn the rules of baseball and American football (e.g., the difference between a walk and a strikeout in baseball or the difference between a field goal and a touchdown in football), he came to understand over time what was happening. He even came to see what was happening better. He could, for instance, follow where the ball was going or who had the ball and who didn't. As a consequence, he went from confused, irritated, and uninterested to understanding the games, enjoying them, and wanting to stay and watch! Now, notice what happened. Nothing about the games of baseball or American football changed. Rather, he changed, but not by changing what he did. Instead, he changed something internal about himself. By learning about the games, he changed how he saw them and subsequently, his emotional and behavioral reaction to them changed. And, it made all the difference.

Let's take another example. Like many people, I suppose, I once looked upon abstract paintings with confusion and a degree of critical judgment – "A two-year-old could do it!" While in college, though, I took an elective art history class and learned about the history and context of the art. It changed my perspective on it. I was no longer bewildered but understood how the art made sense in its historical context. Subsequently, my emotional reaction was more appreciative and less critical. Now, nothing about the art had changed. It remained the same. Rather, I changed. But I didn't do anything different. Rather, I went through a process of learning. It changed my perspective and it made a big difference.

In these cases, something important happened. A helpful change occurred. But it wasn't a change in doing something different. It was a change in being different. It isn't mysterious. The person in each example went through an internal process of change, which we call learning. Each time, the person experienced something as problematic. Through a process of internal change, called learning, the person came to see things differently and they became no longer problematic.

Now, notice where the change occurred. The things themselves – the sports or art – didn't change. Moreover, the change didn't occur by getting rid of these things or avoiding them. They remained constant. Rather, the change occurred in each person. Each person became different. They learned to see these things differently, in a way that allowed the things to become no longer problematic. As a result of this new-found understanding, each person's emotional reaction was better and they were able to go on with the related activity. In other words, they learned how to cope better.

There is great value in learning to cope better.

Like many important things that we learn in life, coping is hard to teach. There is no straightforward way to do it. There is no instruction manual that you follow, like you would when assembling a child's toy. There is no recipe to follow, like you can when baking a cake. There's not even any overt healthcare recommendation to make, like "Take two aspirins (or pain pills) and call me in the morning." Human beings simply don't learn how to cope like that. Nevertheless, learning to cope better is possible.

It's usually done in a trusting and collaborative relationship with another person or within a group of people, and one of these individuals is, in a sense, a teacher. Within this trusting and collaborative relationship, you and the teacher discuss life's problems and the teacher sets the example, offering different ways to look at the problems, using metaphors, analogies, and insights. Over time, you acquire a new frame of reference from which understanding and insight occur. You also acquire a new sense of appreciation and tolerance for life's problems, increased energy, a better ability to sleep at night, less depression or anxiety, and a better sense of meaning and direction in life. In other words, you acquire the ability to cope better with problems in life that can't be entirely changed, like chronic pain. In our society, the most common place to learn such coping is within a psychotherapy relationship with a psychologist. Learning to cope better with any of life's problems is ultimately a psychological pursuit.

Here is where you can see the importance of the psychologist among the staff of a CPRP. In fact, historically, psychologists were largely responsible for the development of the two-pronged CPRP model: healthy lifestyle changes and coping. Psychologists, after all, are the experts in behavior change and insight. To this day, psychologists are typically the directors of CPRPs, in charge of program development, management, and providing day-to-day care.

If, by chance, you don't have access to a CPRP, and are reading this book as a stand-alone self-help book, I would encourage you to seek out the help of a psychologist, preferably one with expertise in chronic pain.

In whatever way you approach chronic pain rehabilitation, whether through participating in a CPRP or not, it's important to recognize that coming to cope with pain better is essentially a learning process. It involves coming to understand pain from a different perspective, one that allows for greater clarity as to how to deal with it. The chronic pain, of course, doesn't change, but you change. You are more empowered: more confident and better able to move on with life's activities. In other words, despite the pain remaining chronic, you are less distressed and impaired by it when you learn to cope better. To this end, let's turn to a helpful way to understand the nature of chronic pain.

Chronic pain syndrome

In the introduction to this book, we defined the difference between acute pain and chronic pain in terms of duration. Chronic pain is pain that lasts longer than six months. We might now add a second characteristic that differentiates acute from chronic pain: its degree of complication.

Generally speaking, acute pain disorders tend to have one cause, which heals over a period of time and patients return to how they were the day before the injury or illness occurred. Chronic pain, however, starts as acute pain, due to, say, an injury or illness, but the pain continues past the point when the acute injury or illness heals because other factors come into play that exacerbate and maintain the pain. In other words, chronic pain is pain that was once acute, but which is now complicated by secondary factors that maintain pain on a chronic course. Let's see how it might happen.

Pain doesn't occur in isolation from everything else that goes on in life. In fact, pain has a remarkable capacity to disrupt life and cause further problems. What kinds of problems? In reality, there are any number of possible answers to this question, but I've noticed in asking this question to patients over the years that there are some common themes. What if you asked yourself this question? Specifically, what are the kinds of problems that you have as a result of living with pain? Do you have trouble falling asleep or staying asleep? How about job loss? With job loss, do you have financial stress? How about stress from credit card bills or unpaid healthcare bills because you're without a paycheck? Does such stress ever keep you worrying a lot? What about problems in keeping your role in the family? Have you found yourself missing out on your children's activities, family functions, parties, or other activities? What's it like when you tell your spouse or children, "No, I can't go"? Guilt, of course, soon follows. Guilt isn't the only emotion that is common when living with chronic pain. Patients in CPRPs almost always report some combination of fear, irritability, anger, anxiety, or depression. Patients also tend to express something more difficult to describe: they report that they've lost their direction in life and that they are stuck, going nowhere. These problems – perhaps not all, but in some combination – are common as pain comes to transition from acute pain to chronic pain.

These problems are also forms of stress. They are what we call stressors, which means that they are problems that cause stress. These stressors can subsequently affect your pain levels in two different ways.

First, stressors affect your ability to cope with pain. Let's assume that your pain remains constant – now we all know that chronic pain waxes and wanes in response to a lot of different things -- but let's just assume for the moment that it doesn't. Assume that all you have to deal with in life is your pain. It would be hard enough, right? Now, suppose that not only must you deal with pain, but you have insomnia night after night. Now you have to deal with that too. In other words, you now have two problems to deal with and their combination can lead to more. How? Well, you are tired all the time. Things that you normally would be able to deal with start to become irritating. Your patience level is low. You start to feel stressed a lot. Maybe you are starting to get tearful easier. You pass on family events – too much pain and it just seems too much work. You pass on your children's school concerts and games. You get down on yourself and feel guilty. Over time, all of these issues continue and you feel like you're getting depressed. Maybe you then lose your job. Anxiety sets in. Pain and life become overwhelming.

Now, maybe, not all of these things have happened to you. The point here though is the following: How many balls can you juggle before you start dropping a few? Over time, as pain becomes more and more chronic, secondary problems come to occur, making the increasing accumulation of problems harder and harder to deal with.

Now, let's return to our assumption that amidst these accumulating problems your pain level remained the same: even in such a case, pain becomes subjectively harder to deal with because you are increasingly overwhelmed by the stressors.

Now, there's no shame in this fact. Everyone has limits. Every juggler finds it harder and harder to keep the balls in the air as the number of balls increases. All jugglers will get to a point at which they start dropping balls. Similarly, chronic pain gets harder and harder to deal with as you experience more and more pain-related stressors.

Second, on a physiological basis, stress can make pain worse. You may have already noticed this fact. It's actually one of the most common factors that exacerbate pain. Please don't get me wrong here. I'm not saying that stress initially caused your pain. Assuming that an injury or illness initially caused your pain, stress can nevertheless make this pain worse and set it on a course that transitions it from acute pain to chronic pain. Even in cases where the underlying injury or illness remains on a chronic basis, stress makes pain worse. In later chapters, we'll review the physiological explanations of how it occurs. It's a little complicated and will take more explanation than I want to take here in this section, but at this point I just want to introduce the notion that stress – in any of its many and various forms – is a factor that complicates pain. It's also one of the hallmarks of a chronic pain syndrome.

Here are the take-home messages about chronic pain syndromes: Acute pain tends to heal within six months of onset and upon healing patients return to life as usual. Chronic pain lasts longer than six months and becomes increasingly complicated by stressful life problems that tend to go along with pain. These problems make it harder to cope with the pain because of the sheer number of them. Additionally, the stress of these problems can affect the physiological basis of your pain, making your actual pain worse. A chronic pain syndrome, then, is pain that is chronic and which is both increasingly harder to cope with because of the corresponding increase in problems associated with it and because the stress of these problems makes the pain worse. In short, a chronic pain syndrome is chronic pain complicated by stress.

The vicious cycles of chronic pain

Our discussion of chronic pain syndromes so far leads us to another hallmark of what differentiates acute pain from chronic pain. It's the vicious cycle of chronic pain. While there can be any number of variations on how such cycles occur, let's take a common example.

Suppose pain keeps you awake at night. As your insomnia continues night after night, your abilities to cope get further strained and you become more emotional. Every little thing starts bugging you. Over time, your irritability leads to becoming easily overwhelmed. This heightened emotional reactivity further saps your ability to cope and you get more and more stressed. Maybe, it's hard now to concentrate and remember stuff. You consequently start worrying that your overall health is deteriorating. In the end, the more pain you have the more stressors you have. In turn, the more your systems become stressed the more pain you have. Chronic pain syndromes are marked by this continuous cycle of worsening pain through the increasing number of secondary problems and their related stress coming to exacerbate the original pain.

Now, each patient with a chronic pain syndrome tends to have different combinations of secondary problems complicating and worsening their pain, but a vicious cycle, in general, is the hallmark of chronic pain syndromes.

This discussion leads to a related, yet important, point, which we'll come back to again and again: when pain becomes a chronic pain syndrome and as such becomes complicated by vicious cycle(s), then *what initially caused the pain is not now the only thing that maintains it on its chronic course.* That is to say, with chronic pain syndromes, the pain no longer has a single cause – the illness or injury that started it. Now, to be sure, the original cause may still be causing pain but this pain is now complicated by a combination of secondary causes – unique to your own particular situation – which are making your pain worse through the stress that they cause.

But don't despair! If this discussion resonates with your experience, I'm not telling you anything you don't already know on some level, right? Now, here's the good news: if you now have pain that is made worse by the stress of secondary problems and, if you can't fix the injury or illness that originally caused your pain, then decide to work on reducing these secondary problems. By doing so, you can reduce your pain and increase your ability to cope with it! It is here that there is an avenue for getting better! By working to reduce the secondary problems related to pain, you reduce the stress to your system and consequently you reduce your stress-exacerbated pain and you become better able to cope with the pain that remains.

Notice just what happened here. You learned about the complicated nature of chronic pain – that it's more than just the long-lasting pain of an underlying injury or illness. In doing so, you came to see chronic pain in a new light, one which opens up new possibilities for getting better. Rather than simply relying on your healthcare providers to get any underlying injury or illness under control, you see that you have a role in getting better by reducing the secondary stressors that are now exacerbating and maintaining your pain. You have a way to get better now. It's through taking ownership of your health and well-being and seeking to reduce the stress in your life.

This is what good coping looks like and you just learned something important about how to do it.

By taking a greater degree of ownership in your health and well-being, you transition from solely seeking acute medical model care to adopting a rehabilitation, or self-management, model of care. You see that you have a role in getting better and it's more than just relying on your healthcare providers to do it for you. Given this budding transition, we must now tackle an important question: have you exhausted all reasonable acute medical procedures and therapies?

Acceptance of the chronicity of pain

When discussing the rehabilitation model in Chapter One, I provided three examples of chronic health conditions – heart disease, type II diabetes, and chronic pain – and listed the self-cares that a patient with these conditions must do to successfully manage them.

Heading the list for each condition was accepting the chronicity of the disorder. Why? Isn't this what we shouldn't do? It seems like we'd be giving up hope. Indeed, many patients struggle with such sentiments and have difficulty accepting that their chronic pain is truly chronic. If you do, you're not alone. I have had many patients respond to me, not without some irritation in their voice, "I'll never accept it! I'll never give up hope that someday I'll find a cure!" So, why accept it? What good would it do?

This anti-acceptance sentiment assumes a particular frame of reference on how to get better. This frame of reference comes from the acute medical model approach. From this model, the way to get better is for the patient to find the right specialist who can fix the problem. Hope lies external to the patient and in the expertise of the specialist and the healthcare system in general. Now, as we've said, there is nothing wrong with this model when it works. By all means, when a problem can be fixed, fix it!

What happens, though, when you have a health condition that can't be fixed? In reality, what happens is that people go through a process of coming to grips with it. This process can go something like the following. A patient with persistent pain lasting longer than six months goes from one healthcare specialist to another; the specialists each do what they do best and proceed through a process of trial and error in repeated attempts to fix the problem; Hope is raised with each new recommendation and then dashed when the attempt fails to fix the pain. The patient subsequently becomes mildly depressed and hopeless. Finding such feelings intolerable, the patient refuses to give up hope and tries another specialist, and then another, and then another. The cycle continues: seek out a specialist, resulting in a subsequent failure to find a cure, which leads to a depressed and hopeless mood, followed by a renewed refusal to give up hope, and subsequently seeking more specialty care which, then again fails. Sound familiar?

At some point, if a problem can't be fixed, you're better off finding a new way to have hope.

Counter-intuitively, this new way involves coming to accept that pain is chronic and can't be fixed. A subtle shift can then occur. It's a shift in your perspective on how to get better. You begin to move from a focus on what specialists can do for you to a focus on what you can do to get better. In other words, you become ready for rehabilitation. When patients come to accept the chronicity of their pain, they become willing to do the hard work of rehabilitation. What are these again? They are regular exercise; regular relaxation exercises; management of stress, mood, and insomnia; tapering from narcotic pain medications; returning to some type of productive activity; and learning to cope better with pain. In the process, you become empowered and confident that you really can live well with chronic pain.

There is, then, value in accepting the chronicity of your pain.

While there is a payoff in the end, acceptance can be a difficult process to go through. Acceptance is an ongoing process that is kind of like grief. The above described loss of hope in a cure and the subsequent regaining of hope through moving on is like what we go through when we lose a loved one. Grief is a process of loss which at first can be denied ("It can't be true... I can't believe this happened!"), but subsequently leads to anger ("Why did she have to die! It's not fair!") and sadness and depressed-like moods ("Why did she have to die... Life doesn't seem to be worth it without her"). As we all know, however, as we go through this process of grief and loss, we ultimately come to accept the loss of a loved one, and a change in perspective occurs. We begin to incorporate the loss into our life and regain a sense of meaning and direction that involves a renewed sense of hope in what the future holds.

Accepting the chronicity of pain is similar. Patients can tend to deny it ("I'll never give up hope of finding a fix! There has to be something they can do!"), and frequently also go through a stage of disappointed anger ("You think I should accept this!? If you had this much pain, you wouldn't accept it either! You're crazier than I am!") Patients also, of course, go through feelings of being overwhelmed, depressed, and hopeless ("I can't deal with this... Life isn't worth living if it's going to be like this..."). As we have seen, however, acceptance ultimately brings with it a change of perspective on how to get better. When you put down the hope in an external fix, you can come to find hope in internal change. Indeed, you come to see that there are many ways to get better by changing both your internal frame of reference and your lifestyle. A renewed sense of hope follows, along with greater clarity on how to get better.

Acceptance is thus another way to get better at coping with pain.

Acceptance is a process that only you can go through. A healthcare provider, such as myself, can raise the issue, suggest it and discuss it, but it's important to note that it's not for me to decide when a patient should accept the chronicity of their pain. It is only patients who can decide to change how they approach getting better– deciding to stop seeking fix-it model procedures and begin participating in rehabilitation model therapies.

However, it's important that you don't go through the process of acceptance by yourself. Change and growth are always easier when you do it with someone. Think back to the teachers who had the biggest impact on you or the doctors who provided you with the best care. With few exceptions, they will be the ones with whom you had the best relationship. Similarly, the most important factor when it comes to change and growth is the relationship that you have with the person who will assist you through the process. It needs to be a helping yet collaborative relationship with someone you respect and trust. The process of accepting the chronicity of pain and going through the hard work of self-management is difficult and people can become emotionally fragile and vulnerable at times. Sometimes you'll need encouragement and sometimes you'll need feedback that you would rather not hear, but in either case, you take it in because you respect and trust the person who is helping you through it.

You find this kind of helping relationship in CPRPs. With the staff of such programs, you can expect to establish positive, therapeutic relationships that help you to accept the chronicity of your pain, learn how to cope with it well, and make healthy lifestyle changes that best accommodate it.

The lack of acceptance spectrum: From reality to denial and idealization

So far, we've seen that taking ownership of your health and well-being and subsequently participating in a CPRP requires acceptance of the chronicity of your pain. If you can find the right specialist to provide an acute medical model fix for your pain, then why bother with coping and healthy lifestyle changes? Acceptance itself thus requires coming to the conclusion that all reasonable medical options have been exhausted. So, how do you come to that conclusion?

If we looked at the research on what is most effective, we'd see that CPRPs are the most effective form of chronic pain management, more effective, on average, than surgical or interventional procedures, or narcotic pain medications. However, we know that CPRPs aren't a cure, and most people, at least initially, want a cure for what ails them. We also know that on occasion certain interventional and surgical procedures produce dramatic results, something that at least on a temporary basis looks somewhat like a cure. So, some patients and chronic pain management providers will consider taking a 'long shot' and pursuing an interventional or surgical procedure at least in the initial phases of a chronic condition.

Many providers – and patients too, incidentally – might consider such an approach fully justified. Football teams do too, of course. With some justification, a football team will attempt a Hail Mary pass, and sometimes, of course, the receiver catches it and they win the game! Usually, though, they don't. The difference points to an important distinction – between possibility and probability. Catching a Hail Mary pass and winning the game is possible, but it isn't probable. Similarly, what the outcome research shows with regard to interventional procedures and spinal surgeries, for instance, is that a dramatic result of substantially reduced symptoms, at least on a temporary basis, is possible, though on average, it isn't probable. So, when faced with the question of what to do about, say, chronic low back pain, do you pursue a potentially dramatic result that is unlikely to occur but possible, or do you pursue a slow incremental approach to getting better that has a high likelihood to occur?

Now, here is where that old issue of acceptance really comes into play. The answer depends on the degree of acceptance that patients have. When patients don't accept that their chronic pain is chronic, they tend to pursue long-shot approaches and, because long-shots are possible, some healthcare providers are willing to provide them.

As such, to the question of what do you do about chronic low back pain or most of the other common chronic pain syndromes for that matter, I think most pain management specialists would agree with something like the following statement: it's reasonable to pursue some modest degree of acute medical model intervention in the early stages of chronic pain if the patient desires, but a CPRP will likely be more effective if the patient has a sufficient degree of acceptance of the chronicity of their pain.

This statement is great in theory, but in actual practice, it rarely happens.

The reality is that participation in a CPRP is usually the last thing that patients do after having tried and failed numerous interventional and surgical procedures within the acute medical model of care. Should this be the case? In recognition of the superior outcomes of CPRPs, many healthcare providers have attempted over the years to make CPRPs the first recommendation in the protocol of care. They argue that we shouldn't do the most effective thing last, but first, when a patient comes to us. Do you know what tends to happen, though? The programs fail because patients don't show up. This statement isn't a criticism, but rather an observation of a fact that has occurred on a repetitive basis within the field. Understandably, patients have to go through a process of coming to accept the chronicity of their pain and if the recommendation for a CPRP is made before they accept it then patients tend to refuse to participate in a CPRP.

Again, it's not for me to decide when patients become ready to accept the chronicity of their pain. This statement is true for a very practical reason: No one changes until they want to. Of course, I might raise the issue of acceptance and discuss it with patients, but until they become convinced that there is no fix, they won't see the point of doing the hard work of rehabilitation.

Now, having acknowledged the importance of patients coming to this decision themselves, there are times when we might accurately assert that some people would be better off accepting the chronicity of their pain even if they don't see it themselves.

The issue, here, is when does pursuing a fix go from being a reasonable option to being a sign of denial that chronic really means chronic?

I once worked with a woman who had twelve back surgeries all on her low back. When I raised the issue of acceptance, she became offended and treated me as if I was incompetent. She expressed to me in no uncertain terms that she'll never accept that her back pain is chronic despite having it for more than ten years and she asserted that if she could find a surgeon to perform another surgery she'd do it. "Think about it," she said, "you got a problem, fix it! Right?" She simply couldn't see any other way to get better. I'd suggest that this patient is actually in denial about the chronicity of her back pain and idealizes the fix-it model approach beyond its limited capabilities.

Please don't get me wrong. I'm not criticizing her. Later in this chapter, we'll discuss the need to find ways to talk about chronic pain and our psychological reactions to it without judgment or stigma. For now, suffice it to say that I'm trying to illustrate that people with chronic pain can engage in a basic human propensity that we all do on occasion. Sometimes, people with chronic pain don't see the writing on the wall.

This example of the woman with twelve back surgeries is a particularly remarkable one, which I use to introduce the point that chronic pain patients, like anyone else who has ever lived with a problem, are capable of *denial* and *idealization*. But I don't want to suggest by the uncommonly extreme nature of this case that denial and idealization are themselves uncommon. On the contrary, they're all too common.

What do I mean by denial and idealization? In psychology, we call them *defense mechanisms*. This bit of technical lingo has entered into popular culture and you have likely heard of the phrase. A defense mechanism is a way of responding to a problem, which, if we fully accept the reality of it, will cause such intolerable feelings that we instead turn our attention away, and refrain from dealing with it. Defense mechanisms are thus the different ways that we keep from dealing with something that seems intolerable.

Psychologists have identified many such ways of responding. Denial and idealization are two of them. Denial is likely the most common and commonly understood in society. You've likely heard about it in relation to alcoholism and other forms of addiction. It's not uncommon for an alcoholic to continue to deny that he's an alcoholic long after his friends and family know he has a problem. Addiction, however, isn't the only intolerable problem that people deny. Parents can do it with their children – deny the reality that their children are getting into trouble. A spouse can deny the reality that the marriage is on the rocks – safer and easier to stay in the den and watch TV. Bosses can deny the reality that something is seriously going wrong within the company. Medical patients too can deny the reality of their condition. Terminal cancer patients, for instance, can sometimes fail to put their legal and financial lives in order. The list can go on indefinitely. What all these examples have in common is that some problem is occurring which – rightly or wrongly – they fear will be intolerable to deal with and so it's easier to look the other way and continue on with life as if nothing is happening.

Idealization occurs when cracks begin to occur in the denial and the problem is acknowledged, but a plan is developed to fix the problem and this plan is insufficiently realistic. It's the belief or perception that something will simply take it all away. Idealization is denial's back up.

The important observation here is that chronic pain patients are like everyone else and are capable of denial and its back up, idealization. The most common example of denial in chronic pain is, of course, the denial that chronic pain is really chronic. Other common examples are the following:

- The belief that you can clean your entire house on a relatively good pain day without it exacerbating your pain afterward.
- The belief that chronic pain doesn't emotionally affect you.
- The belief that stress doesn't exacerbate chronic pain.
- The belief that you can continue to take narcotic pain medications indefinitely without it causing a problem.
- The belief that your life was perfect or nearly perfect before you came to have chronic pain.
- The belief that addiction doesn't occur in anyone who takes long-term narcotic pain medications for chronic pain.

Idealization is also common. Idealization is the belief that a treatment will readily fix chronic pain. The most commonly idealized treatments are spine surgeries, implantable spinal cord stimulators or intrathecal drug delivery devices, and narcotic medications.

Again, these observations aren't criticisms. All people can engage in such reactions to intolerable problems and we are just specifying how it occurs when dealing with chronic pain.

These issues are important though. Problems can await those whose process of acceptance gets delayed by denial and the repetitive trials of idealized procedures.

First, patients can incur financial costs of medical care that threaten their livelihood. I've seen patients cash out 401Ks to pay for treatments that have no demonstrated effectiveness. In such cases, I might raise the issue that they're spending money on a treatment that is likely ineffective, but they'll have none of it, shunning the discussion. In doing so, they unintentionally create a lot of stress –bills, loss of retirement savings, and even the loss of their house at times. As we've seen, such stress saps your abilities to cope with chronic pain and it makes pain worse.

Second, refusal to accept the chronicity of chronic pain is associated with greater emotional distress than those who accept the chronicity of their pain (Viane, et al., 2003). Doesn't it stand to reason? If someone has acute pain, it may be quite helpful to NOT accept the pain and look for therapies to cure it. But if it's truly chronic, the continued pursuit of a fix that never comes just repeats a vicious cycle: recurrently seeking hope in the next idealized fix followed by its failure, with a subsequent loss of hope and ensuing depression.

Third, the repetitive cycle of seeking more and more idealized procedures often leads to complications, which can themselves cause pain and then become the justification for further procedures. It would be fair to say that a large percentage of patients in any pain clinic present with pain that is at least in part due to complications from previous surgical procedures. Spinal fusions, for instance, commonly lead to further fusions because of the strain that the previous fusion places on the discs above and below the original fusion. In this way, spinal fusions often beget further fusions. At some point, the patient or the surgeon decides, despite each subsequent complication, that no more fusions should occur and yet the pain continues and often it's worse. The complications of failed fusions or other back surgeries can then become the justification for pursuing further interventional procedures, such as implantable pain control devices.

At some point, patients are better off coming to accept the chronicity of their pain. Perhaps this book will help you learn that coming to accept chronic pain isn't intolerable and in fact, is often in your best interest.

Readiness for change/taking responsibility for your health

To cope well with chronic pain, you have to take responsibility for your health and well-being. You have to see the management of pain as primarily your responsibility and you have to learn how. In turn, this learning involves the following: being ready to change, being open to feedback from those who teach you, overcoming the stigma that might prevent you from admitting you need help, and developing an observational self. Let's take these steps one at a time.

Here's an old joke: How many psychologists does it take to change a light bulb? Answer: actually only one, but the light bulb has to really want to change. There is also the old saying, 'You can lead a horse to water, but you can't make it drink.' What's behind this joke and saying? The answer is something like, no one does something unless they want to. It's as true for people as it is for horses.

Now, of course, when something is inherently valuable or good, like money or chocolate, we almost always want it and won't mind doing things to get it. But what happens when something really good is actually really hard to get, and will take a lot of time and energy to do, and to get it you need to do things that you really don't want to do? Well, what usually happens is that we tend not to do it. We might give it lip service, but in the end, we put it off. Think about the extra pounds we tend to have. Think about the American diet of fast food and processed foods we tend to eat. Think about the cigarettes we tend to smoke. Wouldn't it be good to lose weight, eat healthier, and stop smoking? Of course, it would. But do we do it? I don't really need to answer the question, do I? Despite how good these changes would be for us, we tend to put them off.

Worse yet, many of us don't even get that far. We might not even think about it. We look the other way and continue on as if these behaviors really won't harm us.

What can break through our procrastination and denial?

For the vast majority of us, we need something that motivates us to make healthy behavior changes. Psychologists have spent a lot of time looking into what motivates people to make healthy changes and basically, it boils down to some degree of dissatisfaction with the way things are. We reach a point at which doing the same thing over and over again just doesn't work for us anymore and is in fact causing enough of a problem that we're willing to do something different to get what we want. This point at which the desire for change occurs is different for each person. Some people, as we say, have to hit *rock bottom* before they're willing to do something different. Others will do something different in anticipation of hitting rock bottom.

The difference lies in the level of denial we each engage in. People hit rock bottom because they don't see the writing on the wall before it's too late. Others will see the writing on the wall and take heed. Either way, we break through the denial and see that we can't continue as we've been going. It's at this point that we become ready to make a change. The problems associated with continuing down the same old path become evident and we come to dislike these problems enough to do something about it.

A couple of important things occur when we break through our denial. First, we stop looking to others for either blame or the answers. Second, we assume responsibility for what it is we want to change. In healthcare, we call this point *readiness for change.*

In chronic pain, the process is similar. By accepting the chronicity of your pain, you break through the denial that "chronic" really doesn't mean chronic and you come to see the problems associated with looking to your healthcare providers for a fix that in the end will never come. Further, you come to realize that the hope of an idealized cure is really a false hope, which masks a true depression. You might find yourself thinking, "Who am I fooling? This isn't going to work. They just keep making the same recommendations over and over again and offering me more and more drugs. They're shooting in the dark and I'm in the dark. This sucks... Life sucks... I don't know what to do anymore, but I know I can't continue like this." By coming to see that there really isn't going to be a fix, you begin to realize that to get better you'll need to take things into your own hands. In other words, you come to accept the chronicity of your pain and you come to accept the responsibility for getting better yourself. You become ready for change. This is the ideal point to begin a rehabilitation approach to getting better.

There are two other important yet related notions: *motivation for change* and *openness to feedback.*

Consider two different people whom we'll call Tom and Sarah.

Tom adamantly asserts that he's strong and can deal with his chronic pain just fine. It doesn't affect him in any way other than that he can't work anymore. Since he's on disability, he's able to financially meet his needs and so he says that he really doesn't have any stress in his life. He takes daily narcotic pain medications for pain and doesn't see anything wrong with it. He's never misused or abused them and he has never broken his narcotic pain medication agreement with his prescribing provider. He thinks of himself as strong and coping well. He doesn't really see any point in talking with you, a healthcare provider, if you can't fix his pain. When you try to talk to him about acceptance, learning how to manage pain without narcotic pain medications, coping better with pain, self-management of any kind, he doesn't think it's relevant to him. He asserts that he's doing just fine and that he's coping well.

Sarah confesses that she doesn't know what to do. She expresses that she feels vulnerable to pain and often scared, and hates feeling this way. She acknowledges that she's depressed and anxious. She's on disability and is able to financially meet her needs, but she says that she wishes she could be more productive because she feels sort of worthless now. She takes daily narcotic medications for pain and she states that the medications frighten her. She hates having to rely on them and wants to get off them, but acknowledges that she doesn't know how. She asks you, her healthcare provider, a lot of questions and readily accepts your feedback and suggestions.

Now here is the question: Who is stronger, Tom or Sarah?

Would it be surprising if I answered that Sarah is actually stronger? How can I say that? Tom states that he's strong and to back up his assertion he points to the facts that he's coping well, that he doesn't have any significant stress in his life, and that he really doesn't need help. Sarah, on the contrary, seems weak. She herself says that she is vulnerable, afraid, and depressed. She readily acknowledges that she needs help whereas Tom says he doesn't need any help! How can Sarah be stronger?

We might begin to answer by suggesting that maybe Tom doesn't actually perceive himself accurately. While we might initially believe Tom, if we thought about it for a while, we might also be somewhat surprised if it were true that he's doing so well. Isn't fear the expected emotional reaction to pain? And shouldn't it be at least somewhat concerning to him that he's taking daily narcotic pain medications and is on disability? So, in the end, wouldn't we be surprised if it's true that he is doing so well?

In fact, don't we already know with some degree of certainty that he really isn't doing well despite what he says? We might subsequently say that being on daily narcotic pain medications and disability, while sometimes necessary, aren't things that we generally consider good. Yes, we need to acknowledge that sometimes they serve a good purpose. However, we can't stop there. We also need to go a step further and say that normally we would also be concerned about being on them and want to get off. Concerned and wanting to get off them is in fact the normal and expected reaction to being on them, despite the temporary good they can do. So, maybe, Tom doesn't actually perceive himself accurately. Using the vocabulary that we have developed so far, we could say that Tom denies the problems associated with daily narcotic pain medications and being on disability, which most of us readily see. Most of us would feel distressed by having to rely on them and would want to do something to stop relying on them. That is to say, the distress that we feel would provide us with *motivation for change.* Tom denies the problems associated with them and since denial so often works, he's not distressed by being on them and so isn't motivated for change.

Sarah readily acknowledges her distress about being on daily narcotic pain medications and disability. She tells us that the medications scare her and that she doesn't want to rely on them. She also tells us that not working makes her feel bad about herself and she wants to get back to feeling engaged again in life. She wants to feel productive. Aren't Sarah's reactions more true to the difficulties that she faces? Aren't they the expected reactions to such difficulties? Of course, they are! Sarah has a more accurate perception of her difficulties and as such she gets that she has problems. She subsequently admits that she has the normal emotional reactions that we all would have when faced with the problems that Sarah has.

The difference between Tom and Sarah is that Sarah has the strength to face her problems in the eye, despite her fear, and not deny them. Because she can admit her problems, the normal emotional reactions that accompany the problems motivate her to do something about them. Not only is she ready for change, she is *motivated for change.*

Moreover, because she is motivated to change, she is *open to feedback.* Her distress leads her to look to others for help. She is willing to listen and take in their suggestions. Whereas Tom, as he said, doesn't think that what we have to offer is relevant to him. Since he considers himself to be coping well, he doesn't see the point of accepting our help to pursue a rehabilitative approach to getting better.

Now Tom isn't stupid. Just as Sarah's response is understandable, his attitude is also understandable. What makes each of their respective positions most clear is to view them in terms of the perspective from which Tom and Sarah see how they should get better. It all comes back to the difference between the fix-it model approach and the rehabilitation model approach. Tom's position is understandable when seen through the frame of the fix-it model and Sarah's position is understandable when seen through the frame of the rehabilitation model. As described, Tom doesn't see any point in talking with us if we can't fix his pain. He sees the role of healthcare providers as delivering fixes to him and if they can't, the next best thing is for them to provide *symptom relief* until a fix can be found. He thinks the function of daily narcotic pain medications and disability payments is similar. It's like what airplanes do when they're in a holding pattern. In Tom's view, the function of narcotic pain medications and disability is a holding pattern which he can do until a fix can be found and he can go back to how he was before all this started – back at work and not taking narcotic pain medications. From the perspective of the acute medical model, his attitude is quite understandable.

While understandable, if we assume that Tom's pain is truly chronic, his temporary (or actually, not-so-temporary) holding pattern is also problematic. And it will become increasingly problematic over time. In later chapters, we'll go into detail about how daily narcotic pain medications and disability have a beneficial time and place but can become problematic over time. For now, however, we can recognize that Sarah has reached the point where she understands there is no fix and is subsequently in a similar holding pattern, but is distressed by it. She is ready for change. The holding pattern scares her. She dislikes it enough that she is not only ready but also motivated for change and she is open to feedback about how to get better through the rehabilitation model of care.

Let's pause here. We should discuss how to talk about these things without judgment, criticism, or stigma. Many people who have read this far will no doubt be challenged by some of it. Am I saying, for instance, that Sarah is in some way better than Tom? Am I criticizing Tom? Many people can become upset when someone like me begins to use words like "denial" and talk about problems associated with daily narcotic pain medications or disability. They hear me as implying criticism. Please know that I don't intend to judge, criticize or stigmatize.

When talking about how to cope better, we have to admit that we are in the realm of psychology. Coping, by its very nature, is an internal, subjective response to a problem. In other words, it's how we psychologically deal with a problem. As such, we have to use psychological terms. Unfortunately, in our society, we still stigmatize certain psychological reactions to problems, such as pain. Let's pause here and understand how this occurs and what we can do to talk about our psychological reactions to pain in non-judgmental and non-critical ways. We need to de-stigmatize how we cope with pain!

Taking the stigma out of the discussion

Let's face it. There's a stigma attached to how people cope with pain. Remember back to when you were a child and got hurt and your mother or father or coach or neighbor told you in a shaming way, "Come on... Rub it off!" or "Hey, it can't be that bad!" Do you remember how you felt? Of course, you felt pain, but you felt something more. You felt something emotional, right? The feeling you felt is called shame. Somehow, and for some reason, others judge how we deal with pain, especially when we have trouble dealing with it. This judgment is usually one of criticism, such as, "Buck up and deal with it." In response, we can get defensive and angry, saying something like, "Well, if you had this amount of pain, you wouldn't be able to deal with it either!" These kinds of shame-filled experiences are what we call *stigma.*

It is the stigma of having difficulty coping with pain.

In chronic pain management, whether it's pursued through a fix-it model approach or a self-management approach, the stigma of how people cope with pain is the elephant in the room. Whether we are healthcare providers or patients, we don't talk about it. We skirt the issue with each other. But the fact remains that the stigma of how patients deal with chronic pain surrounds us like the elephant in the room.

This fact is a problem. One of the two main prongs of chronic pain rehabilitation is to learn how to cope better with pain. Now, many patients are reluctant to acknowledge that they need help coping with pain. It's like acknowledging that the way you're dealing with pain is not quite up to snuff. It's easy therefore to feel ashamed when admitting that you can't cope well. Here is the inherent stigma: society judges people who don't cope well. No one likes to admit that they aren't coping well because they fear they'll be stigmatized for it and subsequently feel ashamed. In response to this shame, it's common for patients to deny that they aren't coping well. Instead, they assert that they're coping as well as anyone possibly can under the circumstances and so refuse to participate in a CPRP that helps people to cope better with pain.

Such stigma and its resulting shame play itself out in my office every day. It's common for patients in my clinic to become offended and angry when they are referred to me or meet with me for the first time. "Why do I have to see you?" they ask, "I have pain in my back. What are you going to do, tell me it's all in my head?" Others ask, with barely disguised skepticism, "I suppose you're going to show me some kind of mind-over-matter technique?" Such reactions are the result of anticipated stigma – the elephant in the room. If these issues don't get resolved, patients come to refuse help that may in fact be very helpful. They refuse rehabilitation therapies, such as a CPRP, that focus on helping them to cope with an unfixable problem because they feel stigmatized by the need for it and subsequently continue to look for procedures and medications within the acute medical model, which fail to fix their unfixable problem.

It's important therefore to overcome stigma. Begin by doing the following thought experiment: say to yourself, "I need help coping with pain" and then observe your reactions – your thoughts and feelings. What would it be like to say it aloud to a loved one or friend? What reactions would you have? If you feel reluctant to do so, or if you find yourself wanting to justify your difficulties or describe how well in fact you're coping, keep thinking about your reactions and observe them, but also begin to challenge them in your head. Are they really warranted?

As already mentioned, it really is okay to have difficulty dealing with problems. You know it intellectually. Why, then, are you holding yourself to such a high standard that you're supposed to have already figured out how to effectively deal with your life-altering chronic pain? Just because you haven't, doesn't make you a bad person. Challenge these reactions to the thought that you need help. Remind yourself that there's nothing shameful about having difficulty in dealing with something. Also, remind yourself of our discussion about Sarah. The person with the true strength is the one who can acknowledge that they have something to learn and yet still maintain their self-esteem. Of course, this process takes practice. What you're practicing is observing your reactions, challenging how warranted they are, and coming to see that it's okay to need help. The more you do it, the more you'll believe it and live it out.

Also, seek out pain management providers, particularly, a pain psychologist, with whom you can pursue rehabilitation strategies. Better yet, participate in a CPRP. You'll receive help within an environment that is both stigma-free and exemplifies the notion that getting help is healthy and good. You can learn from the example that they set. In such care, you come to see that it's okay to have difficulty coping with pain and it's okay to get help. There is nothing shameful about it.

Indeed, overcoming stigma is a prerequisite for successfully learning how to self-manage pain. You'll never learn how to cope with pain well if you can't admit that you need help in learning how to cope. So, be strong. Remind yourself that there is nothing wrong with needing help sometimes. And now is your time.

Developing an observational self

Coping with pain well also involves being able to think about how you're reacting to a problem, recognize when what you're doing isn't helping, and make an intentional choice to do something different. We refer to this set of skills as our *observational self*. Let's review how to foster these abilities.

A common, everyday example might be helpful to illustrate the point. Consider habits, such as biting your fingernails, poor posture, and the like. When we habitually engage in these behaviors, we don't intentionally decide to do them. We do them without much awareness. We do them without thinking. If, then, we want to break such a habit, what do we do? We set out to catch ourselves engaging in these behaviors. We observe ourselves and say, "Oh… there I go again." Our capacity to catch ourselves engaging in behaviors or thoughts or feelings that we weren't previously thinking about – or choosing to do – is what we call an *observational self*.

Most of our day-to-day lives, we are busy doing things. We go here or go there. We react to this or that. In the course of our daily lives, we talk, think, feel, plan, and make choices. We are, of course, awake in these situations and are aware of what we're doing. A lot of it, though, is done on autopilot, for lack of a better word. We get up, say to ourselves, "Ugh, it's early," get in the shower, make and eat breakfast, say goodbye to the kids, get in the car, turn on the radio, drive to work, walk in, say "Hi" to the coworkers and start working. We do these things by rote.

Now, in the course of our everyday lives, we could, at any given moment, stop and reflect on what we're doing, the choices we're making, and the options that we didn't choose. We might also reflect on whether our actions are in line with our values or what we want out of life. Of course, we generally don't. But sometimes we do. When we engage in this reflective deliberation about ourselves, we are using our observational self. Our observational self is our capacity to become reflective. We have the capacity to reflect on our lives and our thoughts, feelings, and actions, as well as the decisions that we could have made.

And importantly, when becoming reflective, we are in a position to make intentional decisions to do something different.

Change and growth require having an observational self. To make meaningful changes we need to foster our ability to observe and reflect on what we're doing. We might do so by beginning to practice catching ourselves and reflecting in the moment about how we're reacting and how we want to react. When we reflect on what we're doing and what we could've done, we create the opportunity to make intentional choices to take certain actions. We might also make intentional choices to respond to some event in a different way, to see the event differently, or even choose how we feel about it.

If, over time, we practice this reflection and intentional decision-making, we can change the reactions and feelings that we no longer want to have. We can change, for instance, our negative emotional responses to problems that can't be entirely resolved. When, over time, we practice maintaining an observational self and making intentional choices, we change and grow.

It's important to note that the observational self is also non-judgmental. When reflective, we consider and deliberate, but we do not judge. We simply acknowledge the occurrence of the thing that we want to change. You might say, for instance, "Oh, there I go again." Notice that there is no judgment or criticism. It's just a simple observation.

We shouldn't confuse our observational self with another aspect of ourselves, what we might call our *inner critic*. We all have a part of ourselves that judges, scolds, or beats up on ourselves. How many times have we all found ourselves hearing that old familiar voice in our heads, "Why did you say [or do] that? That was stupid!" or "Why didn't you say something? You are so... [fill in the blank]." This voice is our inner critic. It's that part of us which tends to judge or criticize what we say or do. Later, we'll talk more about our inner critic and how to begin challenging the accuracy of its judgments and criticisms. The point I wish to make now is that the observational self, which we need to develop and foster when making personal changes, is not the inner critic. Rather, what we'll practice through the course of this book is observing our thoughts, feelings, actions and reactions in a kind, non-judgmental, and purely reflective way.

In the course of this book, we'll use this notion of an observational self to describe how to make changes in pain behavior; posture and guarding; compliance with exercise and relaxation therapies; overcoming depression, anxiety and stress; changing negative attitudes; and even changing the ways we react to pain. In doing so, you learn how to cope better with pain.

Taking responsibility for your health and well-being, revisited

You didn't choose to have chronic pain and you're not to blame for it. However, while you aren't responsible for having chronic pain, you now have it and are now responsible for how you're going to manage it from here on out.

The ancient Greeks had a notion they referred to as *moral luck*. Essentially, it's the notion that things happen to us through no fault of our own but nevertheless, we now have to deal with it or, in other words, be responsible for it. It's a good description of what people have to go through in living with chronic pain. You didn't choose it and never would have, but now you have it and it is in fact your responsibility for how you're going to manage it.

The point is especially true once you begin changing your treatment strategy from an acute medical model approach to a rehabilitation approach. In the former, healthcare providers tend to have responsibility for your health. They are the experts who will deliver care to you. You are the passive recipient of such care. Your hope in getting better lies with them and what they can do to you and for you. We say that this approach involves an *external locus of control*. The power to get better, the responsibility for delivering it, and the hope that it works all depend on factors outside your control. In contrast, the rehabilitation or self-management model involves fostering an *internal locus of control*. That is to say, with coaching by CPRP providers, you begin to take back control of your pain, mood, work, relationships, and life. You don't do it by relying on your providers to do it for you. Rather, you do it by changing your lifestyle and your abilities to cope with pain. By doing so, you reduce the impact that chronic pain has on your life. As a result, you become increasingly empowered and hopeful.

Indeed, through these personal changes, you reverse the vicious cycles of chronic pain. By becoming empowered and hopeful, you become less depressed and anxious. With less depression and anxiety, you come to sleep better at night and have more energy and motivation during the day. In turn, you come to cope better with pain. By coping better, you come to experience pain as more tolerable. In doing so, you take back control of your pain. The vicious cycle of chronic pain can thus be reversed and a cycle of increasing wellness and well-tolerated pain can be established.

Chapter summary

Coping with pain well is possible, but you have to learn how. To learn, you need to understand how you can be responsible for your health and well-being. You learn how to take this responsibility in CPRPs or other forms of chronic pain rehabilitation. Coping well involves a shift in perspective that allows you to see more clearly how to manage pain. By understanding the nature of a chronic pain syndrome, you come to see how to manage pain well, even when it's chronic. You learn how to manage the multiple secondary stressors that exacerbate and maintain pain on a chronic course. This rehabilitation approach allows for hope in getting better even when there is no cure for your chronic pain. To be willing to learn how to manage such stressors, you therefore have to accept that your pain is chronic. You must understand that it's no longer realistic to think that you can find a cure for your chronic pain. Rather, you come to see that the power to get better lies with you, by learning how to cope with chronic pain well. To be successful, you must also be ready and motivated for change as well as be open to the feedback of those who teach you – your CPRP providers. Such readiness requires that you overcome stigma and admit that you need help in learning how to cope with pain. Learning to cope well also requires developing the abilities of an observational self: the capacity to catch yourself in your reactions, identify when they're unhelpful, and make an intentional decision to do something different. In all these ways, you assume responsibility for your health and well-being and come to cope well with chronic pain.

CHAPTER THREE

Three Core Lifestyle Changes

Let's now talk about three lifestyle changes that you should make in order to successfully self-manage pain. As you recall, chronic pain rehabilitation is a two-pronged approach: lifestyle changes which, when done over time, can reduce pain; and, increasing your ability to cope with the pain that remains. We have so far been focusing on the latter prong of rehabilitation: learning to cope with pain better. In this chapter, we'll focus on the former prong: lifestyle changes. We start with three fundamentals of self-management: beginning an exercise regimen, beginning a relaxation therapy, and stopping pain talk and behaviors.

Beginning an exercise regimen

The human body is made to move. When you think about it, for tens of thousands of years, our human ancestors were on the move to survive. They hunted and gathered food and later domesticated crops and animals, but either way, as hunter-gatherers or farmer-herders, they moved all day long. Even through known history, our ancestors kept moving to survive. They engaged in physical work to put food on the table and keep their families and communities going. It's only been in the last fifty or so years that we've become sedentary in the ways in which we work and obtain food. Now, I won't go on about the health dangers of our current sedentary and dietary lifestyles, but my point is that what we take as normal for our lifetime – largely sedentary work and easily procured food – isn't actually normal for our human bodies. Our bodies evolved over tens of thousands of years in the context of persistent moving to survive. As such, our bodies are made to move, and yet, in our society, we don't tend to move much.

Now, when injured or ill, and subsequently in pain, we tend to be even less active. For the most part, this tendency to stop and rest when in pain is helpful. For example, in an acute injury, such as a broken leg, we stop what we're doing at the time. Physically, our muscles become tense, holding the injury in place. Behaviorally, we do a number of things. We guard the injury, and later brace or cast the leg, allowing the fracture to heal and preventing further injury. We tend to rest, conserving our energy. We also avoid physical activity because we again don't want to cause further injury. All of these responses are well and good in an acute injury. But what happens when pain becomes chronic?

Our normal reactions to an acute injury become chronic reactions. We come to have chronic muscle tension. We chronically guard the site of pain. We chronically avoid activities that might cause further injury. We tend to rest a lot. Once occurring on a chronic basis, each of these issues can themselves become problematic.

For example, what happens when your muscles are chronically tense? Suppose, for the moment, that you scrunch up your neck and shoulders, holding them tight. Suppose further that you hold these muscles tight for some time – not just several minutes, but for several days or weeks. What would happen? Your neck and shoulders would ache! You'd also likely develop a tension headache. Chronic muscle tension can thus become painful in and of itself. The result is a vicious cycle: chronic pain causes chronic muscle tension and chronic muscle tension causes further pain.

Similar things happen when patients chronically guard the site of pain. Chronic guarding leads to persistent muscle tension, of course, but it also leads to undue strain on the body parts that take the extra burden. As healthcare providers, we frequently see this issue occur in limb pain when, for example, someone has chronic knee or hip pain and by favoring the painful limb they unintentionally place an undue burden on the other limb and low back. Over time, guarding and limping lead to pain in the latter areas of the body. It's another vicious cycle: chronic pain causes chronic guarding, which causes more pain.

Altogether different secondary problems can occur when patients recurrently avoid activities and rest. Weight gain is a common complicating factor in chronic pain. Patients with chronic pain can gain weight in any of the common ways that other people do, but stopping work or other routine activities, resting, and avoidance tend to also play a role. Such weight gain is, of course, unhealthy, but it can also cause more pain when the chronic pain problem occurs in weight-bearing areas of the body: mid-back, low back, hips, knees, or feet. Weight gain and obesity is also a cause of type II diabetes which can cause a painful disorder called 'neuropathy.' So, here's another vicious cycle: chronic pain leads to inactivity, which causes weight gain, which subsequently causes more pain.

Additionally, different kinds of inactivity cause stress that exacerbates pain. Stopping work can lead to financial problems, loss of role or identity, guilt, low self-esteem, lack of daily structure, and social isolation. All of these secondary problems are stressful and, as we know, stress makes chronic pain worse.

To sum it all up, then, it's natural to react to pain with increased muscle tension, guarding, rest, and activity avoidance. However, when these reactions to acute pain become chronic, they become problematic. They become secondary factors that cause additional pain over and above the pain of the original injury or illness.

So, when having chronic pain, you have to stop reacting to your pain as if it is an acute injury for which tension, guarding, rest, and avoidance of activities will be helpful.

Now, you can't just resume living your life as if it was the day before your injury or illness started! So, what do you do?

Slowly starting to exercise is a good place to start. As we'll find out, exercise serves many purposes, but its most basic purpose is simply to start moving again.

There are two components to successfully starting an exercise regimen: to do it under expert guidance and to go slow.

First, if you haven't already undergone physical therapy (PT), talk to your healthcare provider about obtaining a referral. It's best to learn an exercise regimen that is suited for you, taking into account your particular chronic pain disorder, current physical conditioning, and any other health problems you may have. It's also important to find a physical therapist who is competent in chronic pain rehabilitation. Of course, if you're participating in a CPRP as you read this book, then you already have such a provider. If you aren't in a CPRP, then you'll need to ask around for a therapist who is knowledgeable about chronic pain rehabilitation.

Finding the right kind of physical therapist is important because not all physical therapists are alike. Some specialize in an acute medical model approach to PT. For instance, the focus of most physical therapists who specialize in sports injuries is to cure or promote the healing of the injury. Seeing this type of therapist in the first few weeks of your injury would likely be helpful. It would likely be unhelpful, though, if it has been a few years since the onset of your pain. As we've seen, there is a time and place for both acute medical care and rehabilitation care. With chronic pain syndromes, it's most helpful to see physical therapists who are competent in the latter approach.

Second, you need to start slowly. It's hard to speak in generalities as to how slow to go, given each reader's particular condition. However, we could set a beginning goal to work towards in terms of an exercise regimen. When just starting to self-manage pain, a common goal among patients is to get to the point where they can perform two types of exercise: a) modest stretching and core strengthening exercises on a daily basis; and b) engaging in a mild, low-impact aerobic exercise for twenty minutes four times weekly. Examples of mild, low-impact aerobic exercises are walking in a pool, walking outside or on a treadmill, or riding a stationary exercise bicycle.

The importance of this beginning regimen is that successful rehabilitation requires doing at least this degree of exercise. In other words, patients begin to succeed in self-managing pain when, over time, they engage in daily stretching and core strengthening exercises and at least twenty minutes of a low-impact aerobic exercise four times weekly. For this reason, let's refer to this exercise regimen as the 'beginning regimen.'

Some readers, of course, will already be able to exercise at this level, but for many, it will be too much. Most often, my patients have the beginning regimen as their goal and they start with a less rigorous program. A phys-ical therapist can be helpful at this point in terms of coaching you how to begin. Therapists in CPRPs often start patients in a pool to gain the flexibility and strength required to engage in the beginning exercise reg-imen. Patients start off in the pool because one is relatively weightless in water and so can begin to do exercises that you wouldn't be able to do on land. It's a way to start exercising slowly. Later, patients might move on to land exercises, focusing on flexibility and core strengthening. Eventually, through a graduated fashion, they become flexible enough and strong enough to begin a mild, low-impact aerobic exercise.

Now, at this point, many patients will say that they've had PT and it didn't work or that it hurt too much. However, if you're willing to enter-tain the idea that your body needs to move despite the fact that you have chronic pain because you understand the vicious cycles of pain, then let's keep considering the idea that starting an exercise regimen is in your best long-term interest. There are three things that I'd have you think about in terms of any concerns that PT hasn't worked or that it hurts too much.

First, as we've discussed, not all PT is alike. PT for acute injuries is different than PT for chronic pain. The former tends to be more rigor-ous. It also tends to be more focused on stretching and strengthening exercises than mild, low-impact aerobics. It's also intended to 'fix' the injury. Believe it or not, it can be helpful for many people. It just wasn't helpful for you, unfortunately. Rest assured, it was worth a try at the time, though it isn't likely worth trying again. You have chronic pain and you need PT for chronic pain, not for an acute injury.

As stated, PT for chronic pain focuses on flexibility training, core strengthening, and mild, low-impact aerobic exercise. If you do these exercises on a consistent, long-term basis, you'll get better. Of course, it won't be a cure, but slowly and incrementally you'll come to have less pain.

Second, the most important thing about starting an exercise regi-men isn't how rigorous it is. What matters most is just that you start. If it takes time to get flexible enough and strong enough to engage in the beginning regimen, it's okay! Every day you engage in exercise that will get you to the point of doing the beginning regimen is a day closer to the point of beginning to self-manage pain successfully.

Third, if the exercise that you do hurts too much to continue, then you're doing too much, too soon. When starting out, it's reasonable to expect some modest degree of muscle stiffness and some mild degree of increased pain. Despite the ongoing problems associated with chronic muscle tension and guarding, your body has adjusted to them and any change to them that your exercise brings about will temporarily increase your pain until your body adjusts to the change. However, if the pain that you experience following an exercise blows you out of the water, so to speak, then you're likely doing too much. It's okay to take it down a notch and go slower. Here is another reason why it's important to have a physical therapist at your side. It allows you the opportunity to get feedback on how to modify the exercises. Now, it's important that you don't stop exercising altogether. Remember that your body is made to move and you have to start moving again. It's an essential component of self-managing pain successfully.

Among the many different lifestyle changes you'll read about in this book, the beginning exercise regimen is one of the most important. It has some of the most significant and positive influences on the physiological basis of your pain when done over time. So, it's important to start, even if you have to work your way up to being able to engage in the beginning exercise regimen. Remind yourself that you're tired of the vicious cycles of pain and that your body needs to move despite the pain. Remember too that you're ready for change and that you're ready to take back control of your life.

Beginning a relaxation therapy

The purpose of the first prong of self-management is to engage in certain lifestyle changes that over time will have a positive impact on the physiological basis of your pain. To get this approach up and rolling, as it were, starting an exercise regimen is one of the most important things to do. It's not, however, the only thing you should do when getting the ball rolling. Another important thing is to begin a regular relaxation exercise. When done on a daily basis, over time, a regular relaxation exercise becomes a therapy designed to reduce the chronic muscle tension and nervous system reactivity that chronic pain involves. That is to say, it's a therapy that targets the nervous system, which reduces the chronic muscle tension that is associated with chronic pain. When done on a daily basis, it reduces your average level of pain.

Many patients reply, when I bring up the notion of beginning a regular relaxation exercise, "I know how to relax... I kick back on the couch and watch TV," or some other similar statement. While the different ways that we tend to relax in our society may have their time and place, they don't bring about the level of relaxation necessary to reduce chronic pain. A therapeutic relaxation exercise is different.

A relaxation therapy is a targeted exercise done on a daily basis to reduce the chronic levels of muscle tension and nervous system reactivity that is associated with chronic pain. As you may recall from our discussion of the vicious cycles of pain, chronic pain and the secondary factors that pain causes can themselves lead to chronic muscle tension and chronic stress to the nervous system. Chronic muscle tension can become painful in and of itself and chronic nervous system reactivity can cause many problems, chief among them are pain, anxiety, irritability, and poor sleep. A daily relaxation exercise is a way to reduce both chronic muscle tension and nervous system reactivity over time.

To explain, let's use the metaphor of a car engine. You can see yourself as a car and your nervous system as the engine. You are in the parking gear and your chronic pain is the foot on the accelerator. The more pain you have on any given day the more the foot is pressed on the accelerator and the faster your engine idles. The less pain you have the less the engine idles. Since you have chronic pain, the accelerator is always pressed down, making the engine idle at a higher-than-normal rate. Relaxation therapies are designed to slow your engine down. Every day, you engage in a targeted exercise to let up on the accelerator and slowly, your engine gets used to being downshifted. In doing so, you counteract the tendency for your chronic pain to push down on the accelerator. Over time, your engine remains idling at a lower rate.

Before we go through a starter relaxation exercise, there are a few points to make.

First, engaging in a relaxation exercise is harder than you think. It's actually one of the hardest things you'll learn to do in your CPRP or by reading this book. This statement surprises many patients. "How hard can relaxing be, really?" they often ask. It's actually really hard. It's so hard that you can easily get discouraged and quit. The point here is to forewarn you.

As you practice your relaxation exercise, you'll notice constant interruptions by random thoughts that direct your attention away from the task at hand. One random thought leads to another and then another and before you know it you'll have forgotten all about the relaxation and you'll be thinking, planning, fretting, worrying, or what have you. These persistent distracting thoughts are common and normal when beginning to practice relaxation therapies.

Second, the essential elements of a relaxation exercise are diaphragmatic breathing and focusing your attention on one thing and one thing only. Also known as abdominal breathing, diaphragmatic breathing is a concerted and slow breathing technique of taking a deep breath, filling the lungs first at your diaphragm, and then filling the upper cavity of your lungs. Next, you exhale the breath longer than you normally would, emptying your lungs of air. Then, repeat. The length of your inhales and exhales should be at a rate of one to two, or, in other words, your exhales should be twice as long as your inhales. It will be easy to get distracted by thoughts and noises in the room or outside the room, which then lead to forgetting to breathe in this way. If you notice that you've returned to your usual quick, shallow breathing, just observe that you have stopped your diaphragmatic breathing and, without judgment, return your attention to breathing in a slow, diaphragmatic manner.

The other main component of a relaxation exercise is to focus your attention on one thing only. To counteract the random thoughts that will persistently distract you, it's helpful to pick something that you'll attempt to keep in mind as you engage in the exercise. You need a home base, as it were, to keep coming back to as your thoughts go wandering off. You might try a few different things to hold your attention and in so doing find what works best for you.

The first thing you might try is to simply focus on your breathing. Maintain your attention on breathing in a diaphragmatic manner, first from your abdomen, and second filling the upper cavities of your lungs, all in one long slow inhale; then exhale in a long way, up to twice as long as it took you to inhale. While it may be surprising, it'll require a concerted effort of attention to maintain your breathing in this manner for an extended period of time, without returning to your normal shallow breaths.

Another technique to focus attention is to imagine a pleasant scene that you make up or remember from your past, which you attempt to keep in mind. We call this technique *visualization*. Common visualizations are picturing yourself on a beach in some tropical location or in nature, such as at a lake or in the mountains. I once had a patient who pictured himself in an ancient cathedral that he had once visited in Italy.

Another technique is to say a word or short set of words, over and over again. From certain Eastern traditions of meditation, we know this technique as a mantra, but there are Western traditions that are equivalent, particularly in the form of prayer – the Rosary, for instance. As you can tell, there is some overlap between relaxation therapies and various prayer traditions throughout the world. While many patients might welcome such a common element, you do not need to see relaxation in any religious manner. The point here is that focusing your attention on a word or short set of words is a common technique to keep your attention on the task at hand. Patients commonly use the words "relax," or "calm," or "peace," or, in fact, a short little prayer. Whatever you use, it should be a word or a few short words, because the purpose is to use something on which to direct and focus your attention, a placeholder, as it were, for your thoughts. You don't want a long set of words as then the focus comes to be one of attempting to remember the long string of words, rather than simply a place to put your thoughts. So, whatever you use, the key is to have something to focus your attention on and counteract your natural tendency for your mind to wander off.

You need a placeholder for your thoughts because when your thoughts wander off they eventually lead to some distressing thought that subsequently increases muscle tension and nervous system activity. Before you know it, you'll be thinking about bills or children with various problems or that odd yet concerning interaction with your boss or neighbor or what have you. Once thinking about some bad thing, your neck and shoulders become tense again and your frown returns or your jaw returns to its usual clenched state. As it occurs, simply return to your breathing and focus your attention again on what you have chosen to concentrate on. Put your thoughts back into their placeholder.

Lastly, before moving on to the actual exercise, try to remain patient. Reassure yourself that having chains of associations from one random thought to another is common and normal and that it takes practice to refocus your attention back towards the task at hand. When doing so, try to maintain an observational, non-judgmental stance. With your observational self, simply notice that your attention has drifted away ("Oh, there I go again…") and bring it back to what you're doing – the relaxation exercise. Relaxation exercises are hard to do and they take practice!

Let's now run through how to breathe from your diaphragm. When you're ready, find a quiet place to sit or lay down, whichever you prefer. Pick a place and time when you know there are going to be relatively few interruptions that will require your immediate attention. Turn off the ringers and buzzers of phones and pagers and the like. Commit to taking ten minutes and practice this type of breathing.

Now, place one hand on the top of your chest just below your neck. Place your other hand on the midsection of your belly where it meets your rib cage. This location is your diaphragm. Breathe as you usually do and notice if you can see either hand moving. In most instances, you won't be able to see either hand move. If you can see a hand move, it will likely be the one on your chest. Either way, notice what is happening. Your breathing is shallow, so shallow that you can hardly see any rise and fall of your torso.

Let's try to change the lack of any noticeable movement in this exercise. Keep your hands in their place, one on your belly, just near the lower part of the rib cage, and the other at your upper chest. While inhaling deeply, try to get the hand on your belly to move a little. Your lungs have the capacity to fill up with air down there. Push out your belly as you inhale if you need a reminder of just how deep you can breathe. As you get accustomed to breathing from your diaphragm, you might also experiment with first trying to inhale into the lower cavities of your lungs and then filling the upper cavities of your lungs, all in one big, slow inhale. As you do so, you'll find that your breathing rate slows down. Our breathing is quick when it is shallow, but slow when it is deep.

Now, if you've been trying to diaphragmatically breathe for a few minutes, and if you've never done anything like this before, you might become dizzy or lightheaded. If so, just stop for a few minutes or stop for the day. Try it again tomorrow. You aren't used to having so much oxygen in your system and doing a little each day will allow your body to get used to it. It's also good practice for doing a little relaxation every day, which is what you're aiming to do. Once you've gotten the hang of diaphragmatic breathing and no longer get lightheaded from it, it's time to begin the relaxation exercise in earnest.

Again, pick a place and time that will be quiet and without any foreseeable interruptions. Sit or lay in a comfortable place. If you feel comfortable, close your eyes. Begin to take deep, diaphragmatic breaths. Now, focus your attention on your breathing and try to keep it focused on your breathing. If your thoughts wander off, just notice that your attention has drifted away and return to your breathing, without any judgment or criticism. Continue to breathe, slowly and deeply, with inhales from your diaphragm and exhales that are longer than your inhales. Again, as you do, notice when your thoughts drift off, and bring your attention back to your breathing.

For the next few days, do the same thing, but experiment with different ways to focus your attention. Each day, try a visualization or a short word or short set of words. If you find a method that works well for you, stick with it from then on.

Try to do this relaxation exercise for five minutes every day. Over a little bit of time, extend it to ten minutes, then twenty minutes, every day. It might be difficult to find the time, but it's important. In CPRPs, patients engage in a relaxation exercise every day *for an hour*. It's an intensive therapy to down-shift or down-regulate the chronic muscle tension and nervous system reactivity that chronic pain involves. Having committed to participating in such an intensive program, patients will have the time set aside for them and so it's somewhat easier for them to find the time. While you may not have the opportunity to free your schedule for an hour, it's just as important for you to commit to engaging in this relaxation therapy to some extent. Begin with five minutes working up to twenty minutes per day.

Experiment with the times in your day that work best for you. It works best when you settle on a particular time that you do it every day. By doing it at the same time every day, you incorporate it into your daily schedule, like taking a shower or eating dinner. Typically, we don't have to plan such activities every day, we just know that it's time to do it and we do it. Try to get ten to twenty minutes of relaxation into the same category – something you know you just do every day at such-and-such time and in fact, you coordinate your other activities around it.

Whether you engage in a relaxation therapy for twenty minutes at home or an hour in a CPRP, the purpose of it is the same: it targets the chronic muscle tension and chronic reactivity of the nervous system and over time, by doing it daily, you come to down-shift the high rate of idling that is exhibited by the chronic muscle tension and nervous system reactivity. In so doing, you come to reduce the secondary pain, anxiety, depression, and stress that chronic pain causes. Along with regular exercise, relaxation is the most important thing to do in order to successfully self-manage chronic pain.

Stopping pain talk and behavior

How often does your spouse come home from work and expectantly ask about how your day went in terms of your pain and its related difficulties? Do family activities get planned around whether today is a good pain day or a bad pain day? How often do you get unsolicited advice from people regarding the latest medical procedure they heard about? And then there are the dreaded once-a-year extended family gatherings or parties: the family reunions, graduation parties, Christmas, and Fourth of July picnics. Everyone wants to know whether you're better or whether you've returned to work or not.

Oftentimes, patients complain that it can come to seem that chronic pain is the only thing that anyone ever talks about. While it's no one's fault, this persistent focus on pain day after day is wearing and at times intolerable for you and those around you.

It can cause persistent internal conflict for you. Your friends and family, of course, mean well; they care about you and want to know how you're doing. However, their persistent questions can come across as a subtle expectant hope that maybe today you'll be better. You dash the hope every day because your pain doesn't go away. You subsequently start to feel guilty about being in pain because it seems like you're letting everyone down that you're still in pain. You come to feel bad about feeling bad!

Another more subtle problem can also occur when the main topic of conversation is chronic pain. When you talk a lot about something, it tends to be on your mind a lot. Talking about pain all the time fosters more attention on your chronic pain. Chronic pain can thus come to consume most of your time and attention.

One of the goals of chronic pain rehabilitation is to change these patterns. The first step is to agree to get off the topic. This statement is meant literally.

Tell your friends and family that you all talk too much about pain and that it's time to get off the topic. Tell them that, while you appreciate their concern, you all know you're in chronic pain. While it waxes and wanes to some extent from day to day, you always continue to have pain and you know it and they know it. Review with them that it's not helpful for any of you to be talking about it all the time. So, tell them that unless something changes significantly – for good or bad – you want to stay away from the topic. In other words, make a deal with them that you'll update them if something noteworthy occurs, but, in the meantime, you should all talk about something else.

Now, with your healthcare providers, you should talk about your pain and how you're coping with it. Unlike friends and family, it's helpful to keep your healthcare providers informed so that they can provide feedback on how to manage it better.

The purpose of this agreement between you and your friends and loved ones is that it's a simple behavioral technique to begin de-emphasizing the role that pain has in your life. In effect, it's the beginning of the rehabilitation process of accepting the chronicity of your pain while moving on with the rest of your life. Now, nothing miraculous occurs when everyone agrees to stop talking about chronic pain all the time, but it's an initial step in this 'moving on' process. The reality is that your life consists of a lot more than just chronic pain. Stopping pain talk is a simple way to begin reminding yourself and everyone else of all these other things. It provides you with an opportunity to begin devoting your time and energy to them.

It's also a way to resolve the persistent conflict you feel when having to let down the subtle hope that's implied in everyone's questions about your pain. You no longer have to feel guilty.

A related issue is to begin the process of stopping pain behavior. Pain behaviors are groaning, grimacing, and other nonverbal behaviors that exhibit the degree of pain you experience. These behaviors can keep everyone's focus on your chronic pain. As such, it leads to persistent talk about your pain, which leads to increased stress and subsequently increased pain. So, to keep the focus off your chronic pain, it's important to try to limit your pain behaviors.

For many, stopping these behaviors is more difficult than stopping pain talk. Some patients express that they can't help it when they groan or grimace or grab a hold of a painful body part. They state that exhibiting pain in nonverbal behaviors is a natural reaction to pain.

Such behavior may indeed be a natural reaction to pain, but it's not the only possible way that one might react to pain. Have you ever noticed that people differ in how they express pain? While unintended, some ways may tend to focus attention on your pain while other ways may tend to inhibit attention on your pain. The trick here would be to work towards making your reactions to pain more intentional, which, in effect, is what you're doing when stopping pain talk. You talk about and express your pain when it's helpful and you don't when it's unhelpful.

One way to begin to change pain behavior is to notice the differences between pain behaviors in reaction to acute pain and pain behaviors in reaction to chronic pain. In acute pain reactions, such as when hitting your thumb with a hammer, we tend to immediately react to the pain, quickly pulling the hand away, rubbing it, and saying "Ow!" Might this reaction to acute pain be different from the reaction of groaning and grimacing with chronic pain? Compare the difference between pain behaviors in response to acute pain and pain behaviors that occur after every time, say, someone gets up from a chair, having lived with chronic low back pain for many years. One difference is the degree of the pain's predictability. While we might be careful when using a hammer, we don't anticipate that we'll hit our thumb every time we swing a hammer. It comes to us as a surprise. After having chronic low back pain for a number of years, however, it's possible to anticipate the experience of pain that occurs every time when getting up from a chair. If we know that certain actions produce increased pain every time we do them, we can come to make our reactions to pain more thoughtful when doing these actions.

It's like breaking a habit. Pain behaviors in reaction to chronic pain are like a habitual way of responding to the pain of certain actions. Once you begin to notice and anticipate them, you can begin to make different choices about how or even whether you exhibit the pain in terms of groaning and grimacing behaviors. It takes time, of course, but it's possible. Once successful in limiting your pain behaviors, you can begin to have greater control over the attention that is paid to your pain.

In doing so, you come to have greater control of the stress that all the persistent attention on pain can elicit. With less of everyone's attention on your pain, you have less stress and with less stress in your life you have less pain and you're better able to cope.

When it's helpful to talk about, then by all means talk about your pain with others. But if pain talk and pain behaviors are recurrently bringing unwanted attention to your pain, then limiting pain talk and pain behaviors is in your best interest. It allows you to have greater con-trol over the adverse impact that chronic pain has on your life.

Chapter Summary

In this chapter, we reviewed the three important lifestyle changes that when done over time can reduce the physiological basis of pain. They are beginning a regular exercise regimen, beginning a regular relax-ation therapy, and stopping pain talk and behaviors. These lifestyle changes are essential for successfully self-managing pain because they each, in different ways, reduce vicious cycles of chronic pain by target-ing the stress load on the nervous system. Let's now turn to describe exactly how it works.

CHAPTER FOUR

Making Sense of Your Pain and How Self-Management Works

How you make sense of your pain matters. It matters because it determines, in large part, what you're going to do about it. In other words, what you think is the cause of your chronic pain will influence you when deciding upon which therapies to seek.

Do you think, for example, that your back pain is solely due to a structural problem in the spine? If so, you'll likely seek care from an acute medical model provider who tries to fix it.

If, however, you have come to accept that your chronic pain is really chronic and cannot be fixed, then you seek care from a CPRP. Moreover, if you've begun to make sense of your pain as a chronic pain syndrome, then you've come to understand that your chronic pain is the result of vicious cycles of pain that cause multiple stressors, which, in turn, are exacerbating pain and maintaining its chronicity over time. You also thus understand the central tenet of chronic pain rehabilitation – that what caused your pain is not now the only thing that is maintaining it on a chronic course. When you think about your chronic pain in these ways, you come to see that seeking an acute medical model fix isn't going to work, as they so often don't in real life. As a result, you seek to participate in a CPRP, a treatment that recognizes the need to focus on what's maintaining the pain now – not what started it way back when.

Let's, then, look further at how we make sense of chronic pain from the perspective of chronic pain rehabilitation. It will explain both how and why CPRPs are effective. To do so, we'll discuss the relationship between pain and stress, the role of the nervous system in chronic pain, and a health condition called *central sensitization*.

To begin, let's take a second look at the problems that occur as a result of living with chronic pain. Often, chronic pain initially begins with an acute injury or illness that is painful and this pain subsequently leads to further problems over time. Like what? I might ask you: what problems do you have as a result of living with pain? I've asked this question to countless patients in our CPRP and there are many common responses:

- work loss
- financial stress
- unpaid medical bills
- sleep problems
- anxiety
- depression
- anger and irritability
- loss of your role in the family as a provider or parent or spouse
- loss of social or recreational activities
- loss of a sex life
- becoming overweight and out of shape
- loss of self-esteem
- concentration problems and difficulties with short-term memory
- problems with people doubting the legitimacy of your pain

The list could go on, but by and large, these consequences of chronic pain, or some combination of them, regularly occur among chronic pain patients.

What do all these problems have in common? The answer is that they're problematic, or *stressful*. Stress is the mechanism that leads acute pain to become a chronic pain syndrome – a complicated pain that has come to be secondarily reinforced by the stress of the problems that were initially caused by the pain itself. To clarify how these vicious cycles occur, let's review a phenomenon that is called the *stress response*.

Stress Response

The stress response is our physiological, cognitive, and emotional reaction to stressful events. We might define a stressful event as something that we perceive as threatening in some manner. So, the stress response is our physiological, cognitive, and emotional reaction to a perceived threat or stress.

The stress response occurs in all people. It isn't unique to chronic pain patients. It can occur in all people in many different kinds of situations.

Let's use an example to clarify the notion. The example might be any stressful, or threatening event, but it would best clarify the notion if we chose an acutely stressful event – something that starts and ends abruptly. Let's also take something that is common – something that has occurred to all of us (or could easily imagine it occurring to us).

Suppose you're driving along a residential street and a child runs out in front of your vehicle. You slam on the breaks and stop, prior to hitting the child, but the whole thing gives you quite a start. Now, as you imagine this event or recall a similar one from your past, ask yourself this question: what's happening to you the moment you realize the child is in front of you and you slam on the brakes? We respond to such stressful events in a number of typical ways. What are they? Let's go through them one at a time.

In such events, our muscles become tense. We grip the wheel tightly and grit our teeth. The muscles in our legs and feet contract instantaneously, lifting and pushing on the break. The muscles in the neck, shoulders, back, and even the muscles in our forehead and scalp tense up. We describe such stressful events as "tense," likely because of the muscle tension that develops. Everyday language reflects our reaction to stress.

Our heart rate also increases. For a brief period of time, our hearts might be pounding. We might be able to hear a whoosh-whooshing sound as if we can hear our pulse in our heads. Sometimes, we can feel our pulse in our necks or temples. In other words, when our heart beats rapidly, our blood pressure also rises. With our heart rate up, we also tend to have a corresponding increase in our breath rate. At the end of this stressful event, our heart rate, blood pressure, and breath rate will return to normal.

We might also notice that all of a sudden we need to use the bathroom. We are all likely familiar with colloquial phrases about having certain bodily waste products getting scared out of us. It is literally true! More professionally, when going through a stressful experience, human beings tend to have the urge to urinate or defecate. After having such an urge, our digestion slows for a period of time. In immediate danger where we react quickly, we might not notice these physiological changes in our gastrointestinal system. But, when stress or tension slowly mounts and we have time to anticipate that something scary is to happen, we do often notice it. For example, when waiting for our time to go on stage for a performance or speech, we tend to experience the need to go to the bathroom and our stomachs become "upset" or experience "butterflies" in our stomachs. This experience is the initial urge to urinate or defecate, followed by a slowing of digestion.

Keeping with our theme of colloquial phrases, we often describe stressful events as "hair-raising experiences." Again, it's literally true! In the example of nearly hitting a child in the road, the hair follicles on our skin rise and we might get goosebumps. This physiological reaction is typical in stressful experiences.

We also have increased perceptual abilities when threatened. In the face of danger, our eyes are wide open and our pupils get bigger. In this way, our visual perceptions are heightened. Visual perception, though, isn't the only heightened perception. Our hearing abilities are also heightened. What happens when an odd noise awakens you in the middle of the night? You sit up in bed and listen. Your hearing is acute. A creak in the house is readily heard, whereas when the house creaks in our daily lives of getting kids off to school or making dinner, we generally don't even hear it.

Cognitive changes also occur, which lend themselves to heightened perceptual abilities. Cognitively, our attention and concentration become quite focused. We focus on the here-and-now of the threatening event. Whether the example is reacting immediately to miss a child in the road or creeping through a dark house because of a strange noise, our concentration is quite focused on the immediate perceived danger. In such situations, we don't become distracted by random thoughts, such as wondering if we have enough hamburgers for dinner tonight. No, in such immediately threatening moments, we focus on the threat: it's more like child-break-now! or "What's that noise? There it goes again!"

Heightened focus on threatening events is associated with a structure in the brain called the *hippocampus*. Other cognitive changes in the hippocampus occur as well. With our senses heightened and our concentration focused, our memory is sharp. In these moments of heightened arousal, it's like our memory is taking a constant stream of pictures. As a result, we're able to remember the threatening moment extremely well. We have the ability to replay the event over and over again in our heads. In other words, we can learn or memorize the event in one instance. This kind of memory is different from the memory that we have when learning other things, such as our multiplication tables. With multiplication tables, we have to practice over and over again before we know them and remember them easily. Whereas, in our example of almost hitting a child in the street, it only has to happen one time and it will actually be hard to forget! In threatening situations, then, we experience them once and can remember them easily for some time into the future because our concentration and memory are so acute.

We experience still more changes during the stress response. For instance, we become flushed in the face. Typically, we notice this reaction when people become self-conscious or angry in reaction to some perceived threat. They turn red. Our hands and feet also get cold when experiencing a stressful event. They become cold and clammy. We also tend to perspire. Upon getting out of the car, in our example, we'd find ourselves sweaty and our hands and feet would be cold. We describe such experiences as 'sweating bullets.' Our everyday language reflects what we know scientifically: the stress response includes becoming flushed, cold hands and feet, and increased perspiration.

The stress response also involves a rush of energy and strength. We have all heard stories about people who, in the midst of a dangerous situation, do something with energy or strength that they ordinarily wouldn't be able to do. Even in less heroic yet still stressful situations, we tend to have a lot of energy and the body seems to demand that we act. We can't sit still. We get shaky. In our example of almost hitting a child in the street, we'd likely be so upset that our hands shake and our knees might knock together. In less overtly stressful situations, our hands might not shake, but nonetheless, it's hard to sit still. We don't sit down. We stand, fidget, or begin to pace. In any of these instances, we have certain hormones released into our system, namely adrenaline, norepinephrine, and cortisol, which account for this heightened energy and arousal.

In all, the stress response is the body's reaction to stress or perceived threat, and it includes a number of physiological changes that are listed in Table 1.

Table 1: List of Physical Changes in the Stress Response
Increased muscle tension
Increased heart rate and blood pressure
Increased breath rate
Urge to urinate and/or defecate, followed by slowing of the digestive system
Rising of hair follicles
Heightened perceptual abilities
Heightened focus or concentration on the event
Heightened memory abilities
Becoming flushed
Hands and feet becoming cold
Increased perspiration
Increased energy

Corresponding to these cognitive and bodily reactions, there are also common emotional reactions that occur with the stress response. We have named a few already. What were they? Let's ask ourselves the question in relation to our example. If, while driving, you abruptly have a start when a child runs out in front of you and you slam on the brakes, missing the child, but nearly killing him, how would you feel? In asking this question in our CPRP over the years, patients invariably respond with one of two emotional reactions or both. Most people answer that they'd fear for the child's safety: "Is he okay?" They'd slam the car into park and run out to see if the child is hurt. In other words, their emotional experience and behavior would be driven by fear. Other people in my groups say that they'd get angry. They imagine themselves getting mad and crossly saying to the child, "Don't you look both ways before you cross the street?" Others in the group say, after listening to both responses, that they'd at first feel afraid, but after learning that the child is okay, they'd then get angry. Nonetheless, the emotional reactions boil down to fear and anger. Even in less stressful situations, where we don't experience overt fear or anger, we tend to have some milder version of these two emotions. When stressed, we become either nervous, tense, and intimidated on the one hand or irritable, tense, and grouchy, on the other. These emotions are simply gradations of either fear or anger. Conventional wisdom in psychology associates these basic emotional reactions with activity in a structure of the brain called the *amygdala.*

The stress response is also called the *fight or flight response* because it allows us to respond to a perceived threat or danger in an effective way. Physically, the stress response involves a heightened state of arousal with all bodily systems on 'red alert,' ready to deal with the threat. Cognitively, it involves heightened perceptual abilities and focus, keeping full attention on the threat. It also involves acute memory abilities, which allow us to remember what to do the next time if we ever experience a similar situation. Emotionally, the reactions consist of anger or fear, which motivate us to act in response to the threat. All three kinds of reactions prime us for dealing effectively with danger.

When you think about it, it's a bit awe-inspiring. When threatened, our brains and bodies function together to become highly aroused, super focused, and very emotionally motivated to act. It's the perfect response to danger.

So, why would humans be made this way? Why would we be hard-wired to respond to stress, or perceived threats, with this combination of physiological, cognitive, and emotional reactions? What good would it do? We could add that not only are humans made this way, but all mammals are made this way. Why?

Conventional theorizing in psychology holds that it helps us to survive. These reactions are adaptive when threatened. Consider a herd of deer when a wolf pack approaches. The deer have the same reactions that we have when threatened: the stress response. They'll be charged with energy, tense and ready to go; their hearts will be pounding and they'll be breathing rapidly; they'll be focused on the threat and their perceptions are acute; they might be so scared that they urinate or defecate; their fur will stand on end and they'll look bigger than they really are. They'll have a look of fear in their eyes and in their behavior. And what is their behavior? What do they do? They'll high-tail it out of there! In other words, they flee from the threat.

Other animals do something different: they'll have the same physiological reactions, but rather than fleeing, they become aggressive. Think of what happens when two predators meet each other. Consider what happens in your own backyard when your cat meets a dog or another strange cat. They have the same physiological responses – increased energy, focus, muscle tension, heart rate, breath rate, puffy fur, and so on – but they fight each other, at least until one gets the upper hand and then the other flees.

In these examples, we see why psychologists have dubbed the stress response as the *fight-or-flight response*. Animals either fight or flee when threatened by danger and in a sense, so do we. We get physically pumped up and emotionally we feel either anger or fear or both. Behaviorally, we act fearfully or aggressively. The stress response prepares us for surviving a perceived threat by taking it on or getting away from it.

Now, this red-alert system is a function of two bodily systems: 1) the nervous system and 2) the endocrine system, the system responsible for hormones, some of which double as neurotransmitters for the nervous system. The central nervous system regulates or controls our cognitive functioning (i.e., our heightened focus and memory) and our emotional functioning (i.e., fear and anger). The sympathetic nervous system regulates or controls the other systems involved in the stress response: the hormonal systems (i.e., the release of adrenaline and cortisol, for instance), the cardiopulmonary systems (i.e., the heart and lungs), the gastrointestinal system (i.e., the gut), and the muscle system.

If we had a way to monitor such nervous system activity when threatened – a stress-o-meter, if you will, and we hooked it up to ourselves during a stressful event or to the deer in the above example, it would look something like the following:

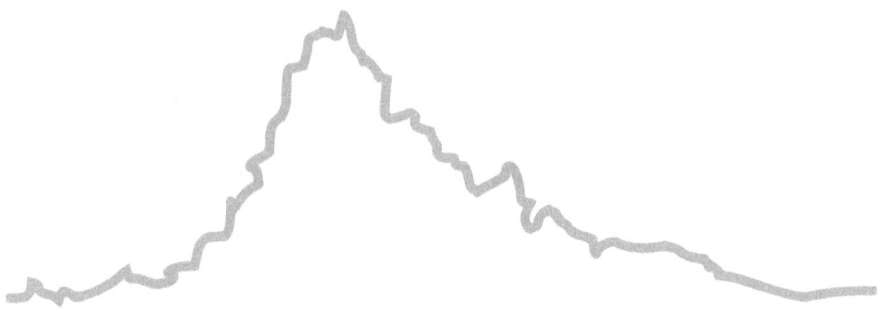

At the start of the plotted graph, we, or our deer friends, are going along with our daily business and then, with the sudden spike, you see the nervous system reactivity related to the threat. It's where we almost hit the child in the road; in the case of the deer, it's when the wolf pack enters the scene. We stop and find out that the child is okay and our nervous system returns to its more normal relaxed state. In the case of the deer, they run away safely and their nervous system returns to normal levels of activity.

Pain and the Stress Response

Now, what does all this information have to do with pain? The stress response is important to understand *because it is also our response to pain.* Let's look at this statement one step at a time.

Ask yourself, what's the function of pain? Why do we have pain? What good does it do? We tend to think of it as always bad, something that must be gotten rid of. While often true, there's a sense in which pain does something positive for us. Pain is good because it alerts us to the fact that we've injured ourselves or have become ill. In this way, pain is helpful. It tells us that something is wrong and we fly into action.

Our body and brain respond to pain in the same ways that they respond to any other threatening event: increased muscle tension, heart rate, and blood pressure; increased focus on the threat; and becoming emotionally alarmed. Acute pain is thus a danger signal to which we respond with the physical, cognitive, and emotional reactions of the stress response. Such reactions lead us to guard the injury (both physically through increased muscle tension and behaviorally through protecting and favoring the site of injury), focus our attention on it, and become motivated to do something about it, such as seek help (through becoming emotionally alarmed). In this sense, pain and the resultant stress response is an adaptive or helpful process when acutely injured or ill.

But what's good for the acute goose isn't always what's good for the chronic gander. While the stress response is adaptive in acute pain, it can lead to further problems once pain becomes chronic.

Consider, for instance, that one of the reactions of the stress response is increased muscle tension. When in pain, our muscles become physically tense and, behaviorally, we guard the site of pain. Adaptive over the short term, but over the long term, if these conditions continue indefinitely, they can themselves become problematic.

Let's take an example. Suppose you have chronic neck pain. The reaction to this pain is for your muscles to tighten up via the stress response of the nervous system: the nervous system reacts to pain as the danger signal it is, as a threatening event, to which it becomes reactive leading to the cascade of stress responses as described above. The response that we're interested in at the moment (we'll discuss the others later) is muscle tension. If pain from the original condition doesn't go away, then the reactivity of the nervous system and its increased muscle tension don't go away. They become chronic. In turn, chronic muscle tension leads to pain! Here, we have a vicious cycle: over time, chronic pain causes pain via the chronic muscle tension that is brought about by the chronic activation of the nervous system, or the stress response.

We might illustrate this basic vicious cycle in the following way:

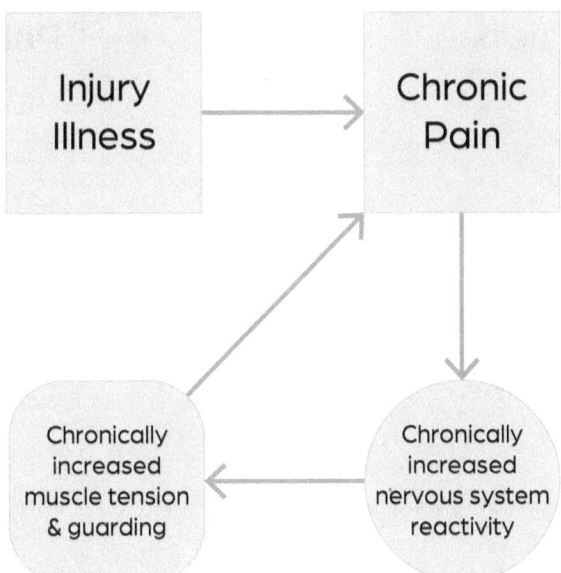

This flow chart depicts a basic model of chronic pain. As we've discussed, however, muscle tension isn't the only reaction involved in the stress response. There is also increased heart rate, blood pressure, and gastrointestinal changes; heightened focus on the threatening event and heightened memory of the event; and reactions of fear and/or anger. These responses are indicators of a reactive nervous system too. Clinically, patients with chronic pain often present with all or some combinations of these responses.

A typical presentation looks something like the following:

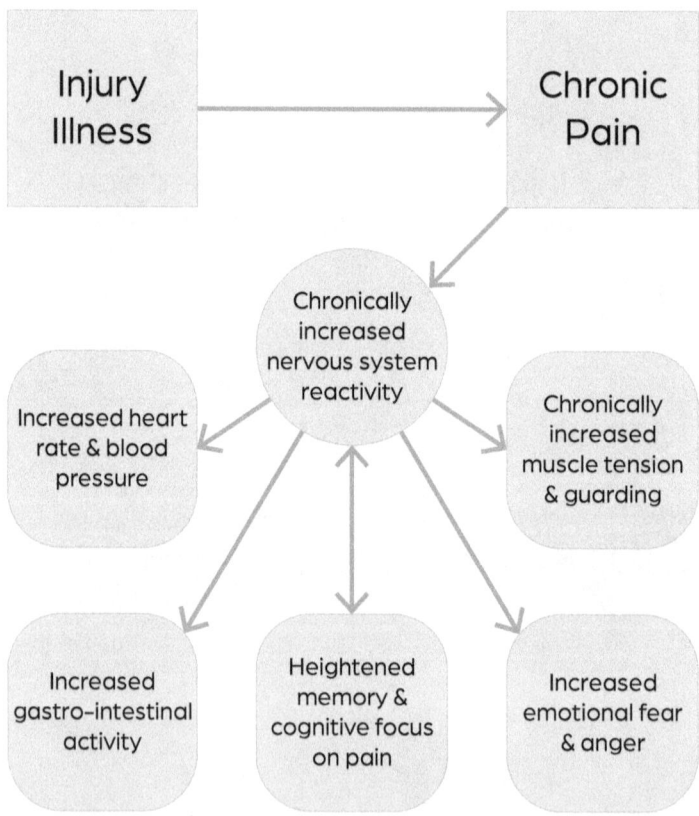

Now, what happens when this state of affairs becomes chronic? These reactions develop into secondary problems for which patients tend to seek care. A typical model of these chronic problems in chronic pain patients is the following:

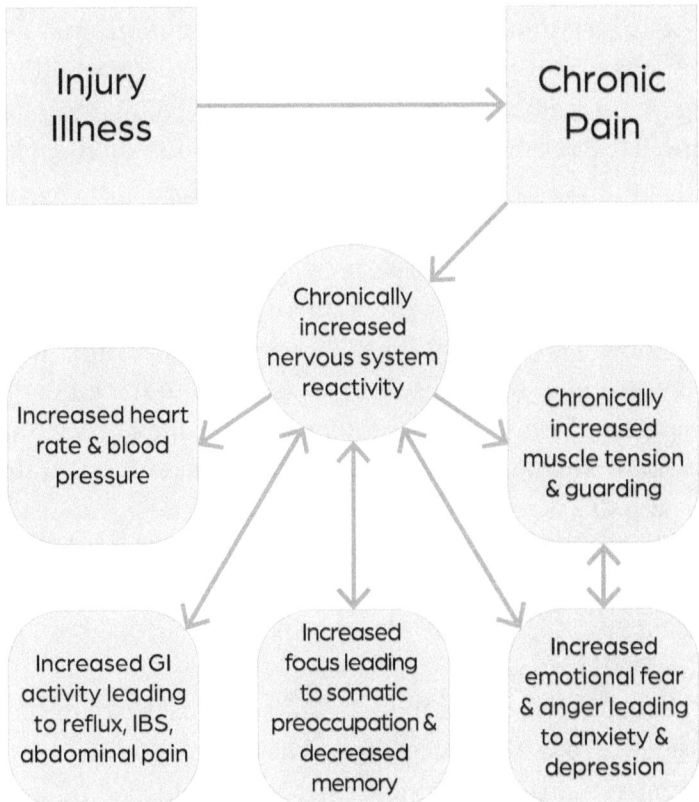

Notice how chronic activation of the nervous system leads to chronic activation of other bodily systems, which, in turn, become problems in themselves.

Chronic fear and anger become anxiety and depression when patients are unable to find a meaningful resolution to these emotional experiences. The onset of anxiety and depression are associated with enhanced nerve growth in the amygdala and a general decline of nerves in the hippocampus (Pega, Sousa, Almeida, & Sousa, 2010; van Praag, Jacobs, Gage, 2000). As mentioned, the amygdala and hippocampus are brain structures that are involved in the stress response. The amygdala, which is the emotional center responsible for fear and anger, gets enhanced, leading to anxiety and depression. The hippocampus, which is one of the centers responsible for concentration and short-term memory, gets exhausted, as it were, and leads to overall difficulties in focusing or remembering anything other than pain and its associated problems. That is to say, anxious and depressed people tend to focus on the bad things in life, like pain, and tend to forget the more routine details of daily life (Kodama, Ono, & Tanabe, 2011).

Indeed, these cognitive aspects of the stress response are called *somatic preoccupation*. Somatic preoccupation occurs when chronic pain occupies too much of your time, thoughts, and energy. It's hard to focus on much else. As a consequence, it's hard to remember anything because pain and its associated problems keep competing for attention. Somatic preoccupation is a common secondary problem of living with chronic pain. It's the result of having a chronic stress response to pain.

The chronic stress response also leads to chronic activation of the gut. As a result, it can elicit reflux and irritable bowel syndrome symptoms (Bhatia & Tandon, 2005; Mayer, 2000; Mayer, Naliboff, Chang, & Coutinho, 2001).

Notice too, in the above model, that some of these problems have double-sided arrows. Chronic pain and its chronic activation of the nervous system cause these secondary problems, but once they've taken on a life of their own, they're simply further stressors to the nervous system. In other words, while initially caused by the chronic activation of the stress response, they exacerbate the already reactive nervous system. As such, we have a diagram of a central tenet of chronic pain rehabilitation: What initially caused your pain is not now the only thing that is maintaining it on a chronic course.

Central sensitization

The vicious cycles thus become clear: the longer pain continues, the longer the stress response occurs; the longer the stress response occurs, the more chronically reactive the nervous system becomes; the chronically reactive nervous system subsequently comes to exacerbate and maintain pain on its own.

Now, if we return to our original list of stressors that occur because of chronic pain, we can see how non-health-related stressors also play a role. In our list, we had work loss, financial problems, loss of the role in the family, loss of pleasurable activities, and relationship problems. These issues are themselves stressful. Their stress affects the nervous system, making it more reactive via the stress response. The result is more pain!

The whole cycle goes round and round, with each aspect – pain, stress, nervous system – exacerbating the others and maintaining pain on a chronic course (Alexander, et al., 2009; Chapman, Tuckett, & Song, 2008; Kuehl, et al., 2010; McLean, Clauw, Abelson, & Liberzon, 2005).

Now, not everyone with a chronic pain syndrome has all of these secondary problems. Nonetheless, they typically experience these factors in some combination.

Among chronic pain syndrome patients, the most common secondary problems are chronic muscle tension and guarding; somatic preoccupation; short-term memory and concentration difficulties; and anxious and depressed moods. These problems have a direct relationship to the nervous system when it becomes chronically reactive.

This point leads to important concepts that explain both the nature of chronic pain and why we do what we do in CPRPs. Thus far, we've been discussing the vicious cycles of chronic pain by which pain affects the nervous system, making it highly reactive via the stress response, which subsequently leads to more pain. These processes are reflected in two concepts, *wind-up* (or up-regulation) and *central sensitization.* Wind-up of the nervous system occurs when the vicious cycles of chronic pain make the nervous system more and more reactive. Within the nervous system, changes occur in the brain and the dorsal horn of the spinal cord. Changes also occur in the endocrine (i.e. hormonal) and immune systems. Central sensitization is the end product of these changes. It's a condition in which the nervous system itself becomes stuck in a persistent state of reactivity, which, over time, makes it increasingly sensitive to producing pain.

Once centrally sensitized, the nervous system requires less and less stimuli to elicit pain. What once required a slug in the arm to produce pain now requires only mild pressure or even simple touch to produce pain. Every little movement can hurt – even simple movements, such as sitting down or getting up from a chair, walking, or standing. This persistently reactive state of the nervous system is the end product of what we have been describing: via chronic activation of the stress response, the nervous system itself comes to maintain pain on a chronic course.

Chronic pain is thus something altogether different from acute pain. It is something over and above the pain of the original injury, such as an injury to the spine. Even in cases where the original injury may have healed, chronic pain continues because the nervous system (as well as the endocrine and immune systems) has failed to return to its normal state of health and remains stuck in a persistent state of reactivity and sensitivity (Benarroch, 2006; Chapman, Tuckett, & Song, 2008; Cortelli & Pierangeli, 2003). As described above, it's a vicious cycle of pain. Pain elicits the stress response, which subsequently up-regulates the nervous system, eliciting the condition of central sensitization, and maintaining pain on a chronic course.

It's hard to overestimate how important it is for you to understand this notion of central sensitization. In cases of chronic pain syndromes, it's what makes the pain of an acute injury become chronic pain. Let's slow down the discussion and relate it back to what we've learned in the previous section about pain, the stress response, and the nervous system.

Central sensitization has two main characteristics. Both involve a heightened sensitivity to pain and the sensation of touch. They are called *allodynia* and *hyperalgesia*.

Allodynia occurs when a person experiences pain even with things that aren't normally painful. For example, chronic pain patients often experience pain with things as simple as hugs or massages. This amount of stimuli to the nerves shouldn't be painful, but because of the reactivity and sensitivity of the nervous system, it is painful. The pain, of course, typically occurs at the site of the original pain disorder. Sometimes, however, central sensitization can progress to the point that patients experience allodynia in other parts of their body, beyond the site of the original pain. In either case, chronic pain patients can have painful areas where even touch hurts.

Hyperalgesia occurs when an actual painful stimulus is perceived as more painful than it should be. An example might be a simple bump. A bump might ordinarily be mildly painful, but it can send the chronic pain patient through the roof with pain. The mild sensation travels through the nervous system, which is in a persistent state of high reactivity and has become excessively sensitive. As such, the mild pain of the bump is processed in the brain as a high level of pain.

While allodynia and hyperalgesia are the traditionally defined hallmarks of central sensitization, we know that central sensitization involves other common characteristics. Central sensitization can lead to heightened sensitivities across all senses, not just the sense of touch. Chronic pain patients often report sensitivities to light, sounds, and odors (Phillips & Clauw, 2011). Normal levels of light are too bright and normal sounds seem too loud or strong odors lead to headaches. In my CPRP, for instance, it's common for patients to insist on having the lights off, with just the natural light from outside coming into the room. It's not that they're crazy. It's that their centrally sensitized nervous systems have led to structural changes in the brain and these changes make their brains' abilities to process sensory information super sensitive. It neatly corresponds to the stress response of having heightened perceptions described above.

Now, sometimes, in my groups, when describing central sensitization, patients become uncomfortable. They hear phrases like "persistent state of reactivity" or "sensitivity" and hear it as criticism. They think the phrases imply judgment – as if to say they are too sensitive! However, it's not so. Central sensitization is simply a notion that explains the physiological and psychological basis of chronic pain syndromes. The terms "reactivity" and "sensitivity" apply to the nervous system, including the brain's capacity to process sensory information. The phrases don't apply to the person. A more ordinary way of putting it is that the nervous system has become stuck in a hair-trigger mode. Non-painful stimuli, such as touch, mild pressure, light, or odors trip the trigger and the brain processes them as pain when it really shouldn't.

When you think about it, it makes so much sense. As the original, isolated site of pain activates the nervous system through the stress response, and as the overall nervous system becomes more chronically reactive, the central nervous system changes and generates heightened sensations of pain. Central sensitization is a helpful explanation of what has happened to you, as a person with chronic pain. It's not a moral judgment at all.

Indeed, most chronic pain patients find the explanation both helpful and validating. Chronic pain patients can sometimes think they must be going crazy because they know intellectually that touch or simple movements shouldn't be as painful as they experience them. Other times, it's not the patients themselves who think they are crazy, but rather it's their friends and loved ones. They witness the patient grimacing at the slightest touch or crying out at the simplest movement and they think that the patient must be a hypochondriac or something. The difference, though, is that such people don't have a nervous system that is stuck in a persistent state of heightened reactivity, called central sensitization.

Central sensitization involves other brain functions besides the processing of sensory information. Problems with concentration and poor short-term memory are common (McEwan, 2004; Yi, Kohno, Moore, & Woolf, 2003; Yunus, 2007). As we discussed in the previous section, these cognitive difficulties are related to somatic preoccupation and the resultant stress on the hippocampus. Patients commonly joke (or worry) that they must have Alzheimer's disease. Typically, it's not Alzheimer's, but central sensitization, which causes these cognitive deficits.

Central sensitization also corresponds with increased levels of emotional distress, particularly anxiety (Chapman, Tuckett, & Song, 2008; Curatolo, Arendt-Nielsen, & Petersen-Felix, 2006). After all, the nervous system is responsible for not only sensations, like pain, but also emotions. When the nervous system is stuck in a persistent state of reactivity, patients are going to be 'nervous' – literally. As we've seen, this anxiety is associated with the enhancement of the amygdala, a brain structure responsible for the stress response (Ji, Fu, Ruppert, & Neugebauer, 2007; Neugebauer, Li, Bird, & Hand, 2004).

With such changes to the central nervous system, chronic pain syndrome patients commonly experience irritability as well. They get frustrated, impatient, or tearful easily. In other words, they have a short fuse and have difficulty tolerating normal life stressors. From here, it's only a hop, skip, and a jump to becoming depressed.

Science tells us that long-term up-regulation of the nervous system leads to depression (Woolf & Salter, 2000). In addition to changes in the amygdala, central sensitization leads to changes in the hippocampus (Duric & McCarson, 2006) and the endocrine system (Blackburn-Munro, 2008), both of which cause depressed moods. Once having become depressed, its associated stress fosters further wind-up of the nervous system (Klauenberg, et al, 2008).

Anxiety and depression can thus become reinforcing factors that further up-regulate the nervous system, which, in turn, exacerbate and maintain chronic pain.

Central sensitization is also associated with sick role behaviors, such as resting (Wieseler-Frank, Maier, & Watkins, 2005) and pain behavior (Meeus & Nijs, 2007; Melzack, Coderre, Kat, & Vaccarino, 2001).

Lastly, with central sensitization, chronic pain can become more widespread (Latremoliere & Woolf, 2009; Phillips & Clauw, 2011; Woolf, 2011). The pain from the isolated site of injury (e.g., your low back) becomes centralized in the brain and spinal cord and now the whole nervous system is involved, and not just the isolated nerves that were related to the original injury. The original injury isn't getting worse, but rather the nervous system as a whole becomes sensitized, causing pain all over.

Central sensitization can occur with all pain conditions. It occurs with chronic low back pain (Giesecke, et al., 2004; O'Neill, et al., 2007), chronic neck pain (Chua, et al., 2011), whiplash injuries (Banic, et al.,

2004), chronic tension headaches (Bendtsen, 2000), migraine head-aches (Stankewitz & May, 2009; Chen, et al., 2011), temporomandibular joint disorder (Lorduy, Liegey-Dougall, Haggard, Sanders, & Gatchel, 2013), rheumatoid arthritis (Meeus, et al., 2012), osteoarthritis of the knee (Arendt-Nielsen, et al., 2010; Finan, et al., 2013), endometriosis (Bajaj, Bajaj, Madsen, & Arendt-Nielsen, 2003), injuries sustained in motor vehicle accidents (McLean, Clauw, Abelson, & Liberzon, 2005), and after surgeries (Fernandez-Lao, 2010). Fibromyalgia, too, is con-sidered simply a disorder of central sensitization (Mhalla, et al., 2010; Martniz-Lavin, 2007; Meeus & Nijs, 2007; Staud, 2006).

If we were to hook up an individual with a chronic pain syndrome to our make-believe stress-o-meter, as we discussed above in the section on the stress response, the graph of their nervous system might look something like the following:

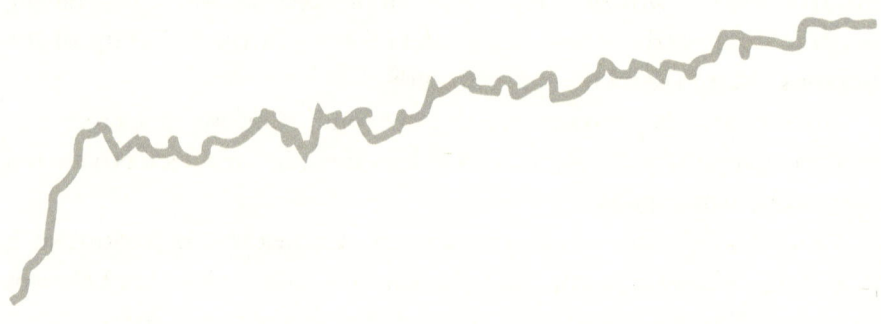

When chronically stuck in the reactivity of central sensitization, the chronic pain patient's nervous system never comes back to a nor-mal relaxed state. It keeps getting higher and higher, in the process of wind-up, because the vicious cycles of pain and stress keep making the nervous system more and more reactive. So, the graph reflects the wind-up of the nervous system in central sensitization.

The power of the notion of central sensitization to explain the complex nature of chronic pain syndromes is quite significant. Patients are almost always taken by how much sense it makes, and they also feel quite validated.

It's not that they are weak, too sensitive, or crazy. There is an explanation for not only their pain and their multiple secondary problems but also why their pain is becoming worse even when the original injury that started it all hasn't gotten worse. They also tend to be struck by how extensive and complicated a problem they really have. It can be sobering. In my groups, someone always speaks up at this point and expresses some type of similar sentiment. Then, someone always asks, "So, what can we do about it?"

Chronic pain rehabilitation down-regulates the nervous system

Everything that we do in a CPRP is designed to down-regulate the nervous system over time. So far, we've discussed beginning a mild, low-impact aerobic exercise regimen, a daily relaxation therapy, and stopping pain talk and behaviors. Each of these forms of self-management targets the nervous system. In the next chapters, we'll review more lifestyle changes and more ways of coping, which also serve to down-regulate the nervous system over time. For now, though, let's briefly explain how it works.

When you engage in a mild, low-impact aerobic exercise, such as what we recommended in the previous chapter, you get your heart rate up. And when you get your heart rate up for about twenty minutes or longer, your nervous system relaxes afterward. You've likely noticed it in the past. We all feel good after a good workout. You have a sense of well-being. You feel grounded. Runners call it "a runner's high." It's the feeling we have when our nervous system relaxes. Now, after a while, this state of relaxation goes away and you return to your usual state of tension. In the case of chronic pain, your nervous system returns to its usual state of reactivity.

However, if you do it on a regular basis, you begin to down-regulate the nervous system. After you exercise, your nervous system relaxes. Of course, after some period of time, it returns to its high level of reactivity. With repetition, however, the nervous system doesn't keep returning to as high level of reactivity as it was previously. Consequently, you re-regulate your nervous system down to a more normal level and thereby reduce the state of central sensitization.

In effect, mild aerobic exercise serves as a counter pressure to the persistent up-regulation of the nervous system that chronic pain fosters. As chronic pain and its secondary stressors tend to up-regulate the nervous system, you engage in mild aerobic exercise that counteracts this tendency and down-regulates your nervous system. You're creating a new – and lower – normal for your nervous system.

While essential, a mild, low-impact aerobic exercise isn't sufficient to successfully down-regulate your overall nervous system.

Daily relaxation therapy is also necessary. Relaxation therapies, such as the one described in the previous chapter, are also therapies that target the nervous system in order to down-regulate it. You relax the nervous system day after day. Of course, just like with aerobic exercise, sometime after you're done with the relaxation exercise, the nervous system returns to its usual level of high reactivity. But, if you repeat it, on a daily basis, the nervous system returns to lower and lower levels of reactivity. Daily relaxation therapies thus also serve as a counter pressure to the persistent up-regulation of the nervous system.

By stopping pain talk and behaviors, you counteract the somatic preoccupation that occurs with a centrally sensitized nervous system. In turn, this process reduces the overall stress load on the nervous system. By doing so, you further reduce the reactivity of the nervous system.

Now, we can add a fourth strategy. CPRP providers often trial medications that have been shown to have mild to moderate effectiveness in reducing central sensitization. The medications are antidepressants and antiepileptics. Patients are often taken aback when providers want to prescribe medications that are used for depression and seizures. However, the medications are often helpful to take for chronic pain because they target the nervous system and help to down-regulate it.

Now, they don't cure central sensitization. They may not even be any more effective than mild aerobic exercise and relaxation exercises. Nonetheless, they can help. Coupled with a lifestyle change, they can be part of your overall rehabilitation strategy.

Of course, none of these strategies is a fix. However, if you engage in systematic self-management, over time, you can down-regulate your nervous system and thereby reduce pain. In the next chapters, we'll review more self-management approaches to reducing pain through targeting central sensitization.

We should add a few points before we end this chapter on how self-management works. Notice that even when successfully down-regulating the nervous system, it doesn't fix the injury or illness that got the pain going in the first place. It doesn't cure, for instance, rheumatoid arthritis. So, here again, acceptance is an important process. But know this too. It's fair to say that by engaging in the long-term therapies of chronic pain rehabilitation you'll have less pain. It's also fair to say that you'll cope better with the pain that remains. With a less stressed nervous system, you'll be less anxious, irritable, and depressed; you'll sleep better at night; and you'll have more energy. In other words, the self-management approaches of a CPRP are the ways that you can get better even when there is no cure for the original injury or illness that started it all.

Chapter Summary

We've discussed how pain becomes a complicated chronic pain syndrome. A chronic pain syndrome occurs when the initial cause of pain is no longer the only thing that maintains the chronicity of pain over time. In this chapter, we discussed the latest scientific understanding of how the acute pain of an injury or illness becomes over time a complicated chronic pain syndrome. The pain of the injury or illness elicits the stress response. The pain also causes stressful problems, which elicit the stress response as well. The nervous system is the bodily system that is most affected by this process. That is to say, the nervous system reacts to pain as the danger signal that it is and becomes reactive in the physical, cognitive, and emotional responses of the stress response: increased muscle tension, heightened cognitive focus, and anxiety/irritability. The stressful life problems that pain causes, such as work loss and relationship problems, further exacerbate the reactivity of the nervous system because these problems too elicit the stress response.

Consequently, the nervous system becomes increasingly up-regulated in a persistent state of reactivity and sensitivity called central sensitization. Central sensitization causes more and more widespread pain, heightened sensitivities to pain and other stimuli, somatic preoccupation, concentration and short-term memory problems, anxiety, and depression. The name for this overall condition is a chronic pain syndrome. It is how your injury or illness – what initially caused your pain – is not now the only thing that maintains your pain on a chronic basis. CPRPs target central sensitization and are focused on down-regulating the nervous system. By doing so, you have less pain and more abilities to cope with the pain that remains.

CHAPTER FIVE

Beyond the Three Core Lifestyle Changes

Patients with chronic pain tend to find the notion of central sensitization quite validating. There's a rational explanation for the many symptoms that make up their chronic pain syndrome – even ones that don't initially seem related, such as attention and short-term memory problems or the fact that touch hurts. Moreover, the notion points to a way to get better by pursuing the self-management approaches of a CPRP which down-regulate the nervous system and thereby reduce central sensitization. Understanding the notion of central sensitization can thus be the start of hope, a realistic hope.

Let's now review additional lifestyle changes that can similarly reduce the overall physiological basis of your pain – central sensitization. These lifestyle changes are the regular use of hot baths, reducing the use of central nervous system stimulants, and overcoming insomnia with the use of antidepressants and cognitive behavioral therapy.

Use of regular hot baths

To your self-management routine, add a nightly hot bath. Throughout history, bathing in hot water has been a therapy to improve health, in addition to being a way to get clean. We could surmise that it's because soaking in hot water relaxes the nervous system. Stay in the tub for twenty minutes or so. Focus on relaxing while you are in it. In this way, the use of a hot bath becomes a therapy. You are serving to down-regulate your nervous system through a daily hot bath regimen.

Now, they shouldn't be a substitute for regular mild aerobic exercise or daily relaxation. Rather, when used in conjunction with these strategies, daily hot baths are another way to counteract the tendency for your nervous system to remain up-regulated.

Reducing the use of stimulants

Pain, emotional distress, and poor sleep all have a common denominator. It's the nervous system. Whatever the original cause of pain, human beings have pain via our nervous system. Signals travel from the site of pain, up the sympathetic nervous system, to the spinal cord, and ultimately to the brain, both of which are parts of the central nervous system; the brain subsequently processes the signals as the experience of pain.

The physiological basis of our emotional life is also our nervous system. Stress, anxiety, and depression are conditions of a nervous system in a state of reactivity.

Likewise, insomnia can be caused by an up-regulated nervous system. Indeed, patients often report that they have trouble falling and staying asleep. Of course, one of the causes of poor sleep is chronic pain itself. Another common cause is persistent thinking – worrying or fretting – at night. This overactive thinking is a sign of an overactive central nervous system.

While poor sleep can be caused by the reactivity of the nervous system, poor sleep can also secondarily reinforce the reactivity of the nervous system. Persistent insomnia makes people on edge. We develop a short fuse. We get tense, restless, nervous, and irritable, all of which are signs of an overly reactive nervous system.

So, pain, emotional distress, and poor sleep all have something in common – an up-regulated nervous system.

Understandably, it's fatiguing when your nervous system produces in you a constant sense of being on overload. We call it the *state of exhaustion*. This exhaustion is manifest, physically in fatigue and, oftentimes, emotionally in depression.

Patients with these problems commonly look to stimulants for help. They come to a CPRP reporting that they drink large amounts of coffee or smoke a lot of cigarettes.

Caffeine and nicotine belong to a class of drugs called central nervous system stimulants. They give us a pick-me-up: we have more energy and focus when using them.

The effects of these drugs are short-lived. We have to go back to them throughout the day if we want their effect to continue. In part, this short-lived nature is due to the fact that our body processes them out of our system and so their effects wear off. However, in part, it's also because these drugs are an attempt to further stimulate a little more energy out of a nervous system that's been so reactive for so long that it is in fact exhausted. It's like a wet towel that you're trying to wring dry by twisting it real tight; the towel is already quite taut but you keep twisting it, making it more tight, in order to wring out the last few remaining drops of water. Like twisting the last remaining drops of water out of an already taut towel, the use of stimulants is producing a few bursts of energy by making an already overly stimulated nervous system more stimulated.

In other words, the use of stimulants makes your problem worse.

Now, not all patients use large amounts of caffeine or nicotine to reduce fatigue. However, if you are doing so, most CPRPs encourage you to consider reducing their use.

Should you stop the use of caffeine or nicotine altogether? If not, then how much is too much? The answers to these questions depend on which one of these drugs we're talking about. Let's take one at a time and discuss them in more detail.

Caffeinated products

Many products contain caffeine. Coffee, tea, soft drinks, and energy drinks have caffeine in them, as do, of course, over-the-counter caffeine pills. How much of these products is too much? There is no hard and fast rule. Some of these products might be fine in minimal regular use, or on occasional use, while others you may want to stay away from altogether. The latter is easier to identify.

Most CPRPs recommend against the use of energy drinks and caffeine pills. They seem to have no real redeeming value to your health.

The limit for coffee, tea, and soft drinks is harder to quantify. Sometimes, you know it when you see it. Patients sometimes report, for instance, that they regularly drink a pot or more of coffee per day. Others report having multiple cups of coffee in the morning and multiple caffeinated soft drinks in the afternoon. These amounts of caffeine are clearly too much. How much, though, is okay to have?

Some healthcare providers recommend no more than two servings of a caffeinated product per week. I tend to recommend no more than two standard-size servings per day. I don't know which recommendation is best as there's no empirical research to back up either of these recommendations. Common sense must inform your decision.

If you aren't a lover of coffee, tea or soft drinks, then take as your goal the former recommendation – no more than two servings per week. If, however, your reaction to this recommendation was "What would I do without my morning coffee?" then take the latter recommendation as your goal – no more than two standard servings per day.

Tobacco products

As you know, cigarettes, pipe tobacco, cigars, chewing tobacco, and e-cigarettes all contain the drug nicotine. Nicotine is well documented as a highly addictive drug and its use in tobacco has a long, well-known list of health problems associated with it. For all these reasons, tobacco should never be used.

As patients with chronic pain, you can add another reason not to use it: it's a persistent stimulant to your already overly reactive nervous system.

Sometimes, patients who smoke say that it helps them to manage pain or at least the stresses of having pain. Such experiences may occur for a couple of reasons. The tobacco helps them focus because of its properties as a nervous system stimulant and so they concentrate better and have a little more energy. Another possibility is that in the moment smoking is satisfying the temporary nicotine withdrawal symptoms that occur between uses. So, their use diminishes the jittery, edgy, and irritable feelings that occur when starting to go into withdrawal.

Consequently, once smokers have a dose of nicotine back on board, they handle their pain and stress better.

Despite these temporary moments of apparent well-being when using tobacco, studies show that when people stop using tobacco they rate their overall stress levels as lower than when they were using it (Cohen and Lichtenstein, 1990; Hughes, 1992). In other words, tobacco cessation reduces the overall reactivity of your nervous system.

There are many ways to stop smoking or using other forms of nicotine. There are smoking cessation classes, telephone support, and the use of certain medications, or a combination of them. Many times, patients pursue these therapies more than once. It's well-known that quitting the use of nicotine is difficult. Talk to your CPRP providers or primary care provider to determine which method is best for you.

Sometimes, patients aren't ready to quit altogether. In such cases, I recommend that they simply begin to use less often. Here is a simple and intentional way to do it.

Take a week and keep track of how many cigarettes you smoke each day. After a week, take an average of the cigarettes per day that you smoke and make a deal with yourself that you'll no longer smoke more than that number of cigarettes each day. Adhere to this limit for some specified number of weeks – two, three, or four weeks. Then, reduce the number of cigarettes that you'll allow yourself by one for another set number of weeks. Over time, continue to reduce by one cigarette along the same time frame. In this way, you get use to doing things with your time besides smoking. You also reduce the amount of stimulant that is affecting your nervous system. Now, reducing smoking isn't preferable to outright quitting. But, it's a start and it's better than doing nothing and continuing to smoke at the rate that you always have.

Improving your sleep

Most patients in a CPRP complain of poor sleep. They have problems falling asleep or staying asleep or both. Many say that they have difficulty sleeping because of pain, but they almost always go on to say that even if it's the pain that wakes them up, it's the thinking that keeps them up. Once awake, they start planning, fretting, worrying, and they find it hard to stop it. We call such thinking *ruminating*.

While ruminating at night, your thoughts are like a pinball in a pinball machine, rapidly bumping back and forth. The longer it goes on, the more worked up you can get.

After a few weeks of poor sleep, patients can come to associate nighttime as so problematic that they get worked up in anticipation of going to sleep. Such anticipatory anxiety further reduces the chances of a good night's rest.

Chronic pain and an up-regulated nervous can thus cause insomnia and, in turn, persistent poor sleep acts as a stressor to the nervous system, further up-regulating it and increasing chronic pain. It's a common vicious cycle.

To counteract this up-regulation of the nervous system, you have to focus on improving your sleep. In CPRPs, it's common for providers to target the sleep disturbances of patients as one of the first things they do.

Medications such as amitriptyline or nortriptyline are generally the first strategy to try. These medications were originally developed as antidepressants, but are usually no longer used as such because they're too sedating. As medications for sleep, however, they're now used because of this side effect. They are typically used at low doses, which would be insufficient to treat depression, but which make patients drowsy enough to fall asleep. Incidentally, amitriptyline and nortriptyline are some of the most effective medications for pain as well. You can think of their use as a two-for-one deal.

As antidepressants, amitriptyline or nortriptyline have no abuse or addiction potential. They also don't lead to rebound insomnia, or the inability to sleep upon stopping their use. In this way, these medications stand in contrast to a class of medications called *hypnotics*, or sleeping pills.

Commonly prescribed hypnotics are zolpidem, zaleplon, eszopiclone, and ramelteon. These medications are often prescribed in primary care and psychiatric clinics, but not in CPRPs.

CPRPs advocate against using hypnotics because they can cause *rebound insomnia.* Rebound insomnia is the inability to sleep once you stop using the medications and oftentimes it is worse than the original insomnia. Specifically, when used on an extended basis, these medications lead to a type of physiological dependence in which it becomes difficult to sleep without their use. As such, with hypnotics, insomnia and its treatment becomes a chicken-or-the-egg thing: at one point you took the medication because you couldn't sleep, and now you can't sleep if you don't take the medication.

Moreover, hypnotics aren't very effective. Buscemi, et al, (2007) combined 105 previously published clinical trials of hypnotics to make one super large study, called a meta-analysis. They found that people taking hypnotics fell asleep 12.8 minutes faster than those who don't take hypnotics. As such, the medications do in fact help people sleep more – but not by much more.

For an average of 13 more minutes of sleep per night, are hypnotics worth the risk of becoming dependent on them and unable to sleep without them?

If you're someone who has been taking a hypnotic on a chronic basis, you might want to talk with your CPRP providers about attempting to manage your insomnia in a more effective way. A typical CPRP treatment plan for insomnia is to slowly taper hypnotics as directed by a healthcare provider, possibly using an antidepressant to help, such as amitriptyline or nortriptyline, and to pursue cognitive behavior therapies, sleep hygiene, and exercise. Let's take these one at a time because whether taking a hypnotic or not, if you have insomnia, these strategies are the most helpful therapies to pursue.

Cognitive behavior therapy (CBT) is a treatment used for chronic pain, insomnia, anxiety, depression, and other problems. We'll go into many CBT principles in later chapters. For now, let's focus on CBT as it relates to insomnia.

The first thing to do is to practice developing an observational self. You may recall from Chapter Two, your observational self is the ability to observe yourself in any given situation and think about how you're reacting to the situation.

You can begin to practice your abilities to observe yourself in two ways. First, begin to observe your anticipatory reactions – thoughts and feelings – about going to bed. Second, begin to observe your ruminative thoughts when lying awake at night. Think of your anticipatory apprehensions and the ruminative thoughts as habits of thinking – habitual ways of reacting to going to bed and habitual ways of thinking while awake at night. Like any habit, we often start fretting and ruminating without much consideration that we're doing it. It just sort of happens and we get increasingly worked up. We can, however, set out to observe and catch ourselves doing it. It's the first thing to do when breaking any bad habit. You catch yourself doing it and bring greater awareness to it.

Once you are catching yourself having these thoughts and feelings, try to make the choice to do something different. For example, begin diaphragmatically breathing or if you're already in bed, start your relaxation exercise. As you fall back into your habitual rumination, catch yourself and make a mental note that you're doing it. Practice making the choice to bring your attention back to the relaxation exercise. Each time you slip, catch yourself, observe it, and attempt to make a choice to engage in diaphragmatic breathing. Do it over and over again.

Try not to get too frustrated with yourself. Breaking a habit – any habit – is hard to do and takes a lot of practice. Don't expect that you'll easily be able to keep yourself from falling back into thinking about troublesome things at night. So, don't set the bar too high. Expect that it's going to take practice and coaching from your CPRP staff.

Once you begin catching yourself in the habitual apprehensions and ruminations that keep you awake, it's time to begin making the decision to challenge them. You'll do so by engaging in a set of behavior changes called *sleep restriction* and *stimulus control*. They are the principal components of CBT for insomnia.

In general, sleep restriction involves limiting the amount of time spent in bed to only the time spent sleeping. In other words, don't lie in bed if you're not sleeping.

Specifically, pick a reasonable time to go to bed at night and a reasonable time to get up in the morning. For most adults, there should be about six to eight hours between the time you go to bed and the time you get out of bed. Preferably, these six to eight hours should be at night.

Now, start going to bed at the same time every night, within reason. If you're not sleepy, get out of bed and leave the bedroom. Spend time with a quiet, non-stimulating activity (see the paragraph below on sleep hygiene), such as reading, knitting, doing a puzzle, or listening to relaxing music until you're sleepy. Once sleepy, go back to bed and try to fall asleep. Repeat this process as needed.

By doing this practice, you restrict the time spent in bed that you're not sleeping. In other words, you interrupt the habit of ruminating in bed.

Now, you also must restrict yourself from sleeping outside the six to eight hour time frame that you committed to sleeping. No matter how little you slept the night before, you are to still wake up and get out of bed at your scheduled wake-up time. Moreover, you must remain awake throughout the day, intentionally refusing to nap. To do so, distract yourself by engaging in your usual activities and keeping your usual routines.

Of course, you may have some days in which you are really tired. You also might not be very productive during these days. Rest assured, though. Your daytime tiredness is temporary because you're engaged in effective changes that will lead to success.

You are making both physical changes and psychological changes that will over time help you to sleep better on a regular basis. This goal is a big win that is worth the temporary discomfort of being tired when you initially start this process of getting up at the same time every day and refusing to nap during the day, despite poor sleep.

First, you are changing your *circadian rhythm*. Circadian rhythm is a term that refers to the body's 'clock,' which regulates sleepiness and wakefulness. It is an environmental and biochemical process that leads us to naturally become sleepy at night and naturally start waking up in the morning.

While it's a bodily process, it is altered by environmental and behavioral factors. The most important environmental factor is light. The light-dark cycle of sunlight, going from day to night over and over again, alters and, in fact, regulates our circadian rhythm. The other most important factor is our own behavior. As we know from shift workers, humans can 'override' the natural regulation that day and night produces and people can come to the point of changing their sleep-wake cycle to some extent.

Habitual anticipatory anxiety prior to bed and ruminations at night can also re-regulate the circadian rhythm. These manifestations of an over-reactive nervous system keep you awake at night and then behaviorally you respond to your poor night's sleep by napping during the day. If you engage in these behaviors repetitively, you alter your circadian rhythm and tend towards wakefulness at night and sleepiness during the day.

One good way to change this alteration in the body's sleep-wake clock is to behaviorally override it and use the natural light-dark cycle as your ally. In other words, what you do is what we described above: You pick a reasonable amount of time (6-8 hours at night) to sleep; try to sleep, but if you can't, get up and engage in a quiet repetitive activity, and return to bed when sleepy; get up at your agreed upon time in the morning – no matter how much or little you slept; and remain awake until your agreed upon time to return to sleep at night. Over time, you re-regulate your circadian rhythm – the body's natural sleep-wake cycle.

Second, in committing to these behavioral changes, you make an important psychological change. Specifically, you break the habits of thinking that can impair sleep so much – the anticipatory anxiety when you go to bed and the rumination that occurs while awake at night. How does this occur?

One way to explain it is to first recognize that we're all creatures of habit. We all have our habits that we do at certain times of the day, in response to certain things, people, or events. In psychology, we call such habits *associations* because the habitual things we do are associated with certain times, events, places, or things. To take a simple example, many of us lived the first twenty or so years of our lives without ever thinking about drinking coffee in the morning. But at some point, usually in young adulthood, we were introduced to coffee in the morning and over time we became morning coffee drinkers. Now, it might be hard to imagine a morning without a cup. We've developed a habit of drinking coffee in the morning through the persistent association of drinking it at a certain time of the day. Lo and behold, if we tried to stop drinking coffee, the hardest time of our day to go without it would be in the morning. It's because we've come to associate the morning with having coffee. The same can be true with any other habit.

In the habitual ways of thinking that disrupt sleep, the same process of association has occurred. Whether it's anticipatory apprehension of going to sleep or rumination while lying in bed, we have come to associate the time (i.e., bedtime) or place (i.e., the bed or bedroom) with these habitual ways of thinking. As a result, it's hard to stop these ways of thinking at this time and place – nighttime in your bedroom.

The best way to break a habit is to expose yourself to a new activity in a new place when you observe yourself engaged in the habit. In this case, the habits are apprehensions and ruminations. So, if you can't sleep and you catch yourself apprehensively ruminating, re-direct your attention by getting out of bed and engaging in a quiet repetitive activity, such as reading or knitting, until you're tired and then return to bed. By exposing yourself to a new thing in a new place each time you begin to ruminate, you break the association that you have between being in bed and ruminating. As you practice it over time, you come to associate bedtime with sleepiness, rather than worries.

What we just described is a process that we earlier referred to as stimulus control. You change your associations of going to bed or being in bed by controlling the stimulus with which you develop these associations. Each time you stop lying in bed while fretting, and instead get up to do something different, and each time you go back to bed only when you're sleepy, you engage in stimulus control. Over time, you no longer anticipate insomnia or fret and worry. Rather, you associate going to bed with sleepiness.

To further this process, it helps to improve your *sleep hygiene.* This phrase refers to making healthy changes in your activities and your immediate environment to improve sleep. Let's review both.

First, stop watching television at least an hour before bedtime. This recommendation is hard for many people to make. We often think of watching television as relaxing – "I'm going to kick back and watch some TV," one might say. In actuality, though, television doesn't relax us. TV shows are enjoyable and hold our attention because they are stimulating. Think about it. What do we tend to watch? Comedies, suspenseful thrillers, murder mysteries, game shows, shows with sexual themes, and news or talk shows about politics. How do these shows hold our attention? They do so by stimulating us – we laugh (i.e., the comedies), get thrilled (i.e., suspense shows), excited (i.e., game shows), aroused (i.e., sex scenes), disturbed (i.e., the news), or impassioned (i.e., political talk shows). None of these forms of stimulation is actually conducive to sleep. When you stop watching television an hour or more before bedtime, you provide your nervous system an opportunity to wind down.

Now, some patients report at this point that they find it helpful to have the television on at night in the bedroom as they fall asleep and even while they stay asleep. Such a habit shows how you can get used to the up-regulation of the nervous system.

Suppose for the moment that we aren't talking about chronic pain and the chronic up-regulation of the nervous system that goes with it. Rather, we're just talking about the habit of having the television on while going to sleep. If we're in agreement that television is at least modestly stimulating, how does someone get used to such stimulation when falling asleep? Doesn't it seem odd?

A similar example is the effect that the white noise of a fan has on us over time. At first, when we turn the fan on, it seems loud, but over time we fail to notice it any longer. Despite getting used to it, the loud sound continues and it continues to affect our nervous system, making our muscles tense. We aren't aware of this subtle up-regulation of our nervous system until we turn the fan off and experience the relief that we have. We automatically notice it and our muscles relax! We realize that we weren't aware of the 'new normal' that the constant white noise of the fan had produced. In effect, this new normal was a mini up-regulation of our nervous system.

The same thing happens when patients have the television on as they fall or stay asleep. They maintain the new normal of the up-regulation of the nervous system.

So, when turning off the television, it might feel abnormal. However, it's what a more relaxed nervous system feels like! Now, simply stopping TV watching won't down-regulate the nervous system by itself. What you're doing, though, is stopping the addition of a modest amount of fuel to the fire. You're also increasing the opportunity that you'll sleep more soundly.

Next, establish a new bedtime routine. First, do things that lend themselves to winding down and relaxing. Second, do these things in approximately the same order each night. For instance, suppose each night you take a hot bath, get into your pajamas, and read for an hour. Maybe you get a warm blanket, curl up with your dog or cat, and journal each night. Of course, you'll want to do things that align with your interests but focus on things that are relaxing. As you do them in roughly the same order each night, you create new associations to which you train your nervous system to wind down.

Avoid alcohol use. It may help you to fall asleep, but once the alcohol is processed out of your system, you'll experience a rebound of light sleep and you may in fact wake up altogether. So, in the end, you'll lose quality and quantity sleep.

Also, follow the above guidelines on the use of caffeinated beverages. It might go without saying, but a surprisingly large number of people report drinking coffee late into the afternoon or evening, despite having insomnia. It's one of the many vicious cycles that chronic pain can generate: chronic pain causes insomnia, which results in fatigue to which patients respond with caffeinated beverage use. While understandable, the only way out of this cycle is through it, by reducing caffeinated beverage use and putting up with the fatigue during the day.

Lastly, begin an exercise regimen as described in Chapter Three. We already reviewed how the body is made to move. But, it's also made to sleep. The two are connected. When you exercise during the day, you'll naturally sleep better at night.

As you make all these changes, you may notice the emergence of a new cycle, not a vicious cycle but a beneficial cycle. You've begun regular exercise and relaxation regimes and over a few weeks you begin to notice that you're sleeping better, but you've also made healthy changes in your sleeping habits and so have begun to have restful sleep more frequently; consequently, you have more energy and a better outlook. As this beneficial cycle continues, the more down-regulated your nervous system becomes. As a result, you have less pain and stress, and become better able to cope, which are your goals.

Chapter Summary

You're beginning to take back control. Hopefully, you have found a CPRP in your area and have sought their assistance. If you don't have a program in your area, hopefully, you've found a chronic pain rehabilitation provider to see on a regular basis. Either way, by now, you have an understanding of the complexity of your pain disorder: while you may have a health condition that causes ongoing pain, you also have a more widespread nervous system problem in terms of central sensitization that is exacerbating and maintaining the chronicity of your pain. This up-regulation of the nervous system has both physical and emotional symptoms. It's like a coin with pain on one side and emotional distress on the other.

However, you understand that the way to get better is not to fix the original problem – you've tried that and have exhausted all reasonable options. Rather, you understand that to get better you need to down-regulate the nervous system.

You've begun regular exercise and relaxation regimens. You take a daily hot bath. You're reducing or stopping the use of caffeinated products and/or tobacco products. You're making healthy changes in your sleep habits by refusing to nap, challenging your ruminations by establishing new associations, and creating a bedtime routine.

The more you make each of these changes, the easier it gets to make the others. The more exercise you get, the more relaxation you pursue, and the less caffeine or nicotine you use, the better you sleep. The better you sleep, the more energy and motivation you have and the brighter your mood is. In turn, your brighter outlook leads to budding confidence and motivation to continue these healthy changes.

You begin, then, a beneficial cycle that down-regulates your nervous system and you subsequently come to have less pain and stress. Get excited about the possibility of hope again. You're establishing an internal locus of control and taking responsibility for your health. Your perspective is shifting to a renewed confidence that change is possible and is in fact underway.

CHAPTER SIX

Overcoming the Stressors
of Living with Chronic Pain

In the previous chapter, we discussed various ways to pursue the first prong of self-management: making lifestyle changes that reduce the central sensitization that is at least partially (if not wholly) the physiological basis of your pain. It's time now to return to a discussion of how to pursue the second prong of self-management: ways to cope with the pain that remains.

Coping is our subjective response to a problem

There's no easy way to teach people how to cope better with a problem. As we've said, we don't have any instruction manuals for it. It's probably because coping isn't really about doing things differently. It's about being different. It's about approaching a problem differently by adopting a new perspective on the problem. It's an internal process that occurs when dealing with an external problem.

While there is no recipe to follow, what we do in CPRPs is that we start to talk about it, describe it, envision it, and at some point patients begin to 'catch on.' They start seeing their problems differently – as not so problematic. They realize that they are subtly changing. They no longer see themselves as so helpless or angry or stressed by pain. They're more open to getting back into life. They've become more confident. Let's start talking about seeing your problems in this light.

I want to make a point before we continue. This section clarifies the notion of coping and it's one of the most important parts of this book. By understanding what's described here, you open up a whole new way to get better. The ramifications are great. The remainder of this book builds on the understanding that comes from this section.

To begin, let's talk about coping in general so that we get our bearings and then proceed to specific ways to cope better that we know are effective.

What does the word "coping" really mean? In general, we might define "coping" as the way we deal with a problem. It's the way we react to or respond to a problem in order to overcome it. We should discuss three important aspects of coping.

First, we typically consider it a subjective experience. Coping is an internal way we react to problems. How we cope with a problem is dependent on how we see the problem, the perspective that we take on it, how we make sense of the problem, how we emotionally react to it, and so on. Other factors that determine how we react to a problem are whether we've dealt with the problem before or how well-practiced we are in dealing with it. What others have taught us about a problem and how to deal with it plays a role too. Sometimes, people have explicitly taught us about a problem and how to respond to it. Other times, we have had coping responses simply role-modeled for us.

You might notice that all these factors are psychological in nature and so we typically think of coping as a subjective or internal response to a problem. Now, the problems themselves may be internal difficulties, such as anxiety, depression, or insomnia, or external problems, such as the death of a loved one or a natural disaster. Whatever the problem, coping is an internal or subjective way of responding to the problem in order to deal with it. It's essentially a psychological process.

Second, there is a range of ways that people cope with any specific problem. People can look upon the same problem differently, make sense of it differently, and subsequently have different emotional reactions in their attempts to overcome it. Some are ill-prepared to deal with the problem and some are well-prepared. Despite these common differences, there are also typical ways that we all respond to problems. There are common themes, as it were, on how we deal with problems. Psychologists have identified them and given names to them. In a moment, we'll review some of them, seeing how some ways of coping usually work well while other ones are often not so successful. This point brings us to our last important aspect of coping.

Third, in this range of coping responses, some work better than others. We identify these differences in coping across different individuals – some people cope better than others with the same problem. One person might cope with a stressful problem by drinking too much while another person might respond to the same problem with exercise as a way to feel better. In other instances, we might notice that an individual comes to cope better or worse with a problem over time. So, one person at a particular time in her life might have responded to a stressful day at work with a stop at the liquor store on the way home while later in life she might go for a walk after work. We might therefore state that coping can be seen as occurring along a spectrum from better to worse.

We might sum up our three general statements about coping: 1) coping is a subjective, or psychological, response to a problem; 2) how we cope with a problem can differ from person to person or from time to time, but there are common ways that we all cope with problems as well; and 3) we can cope better or worse with problems.

We could represent these three aspects in the following illustration.

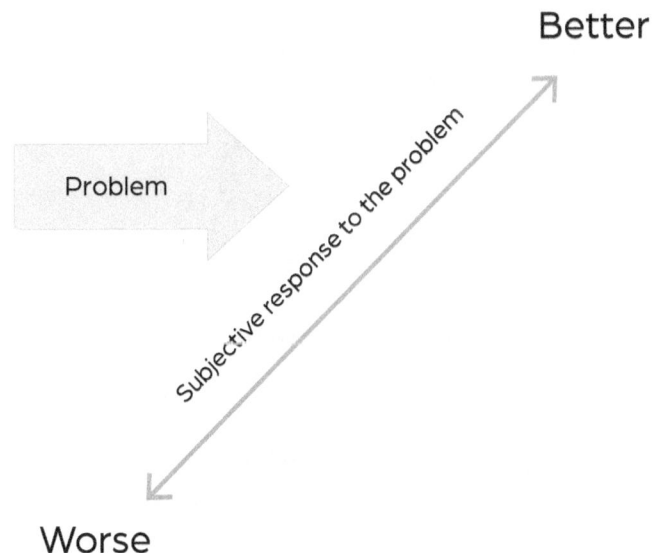

The large, thick arrow to the left represents a problem and the thinner, tilted arrow in the middle represents the spectrum of possible ways that we might cope with the problem.

In the example above, regarding how a person copes with a stressful day at work, we might use this illustration to represent it.

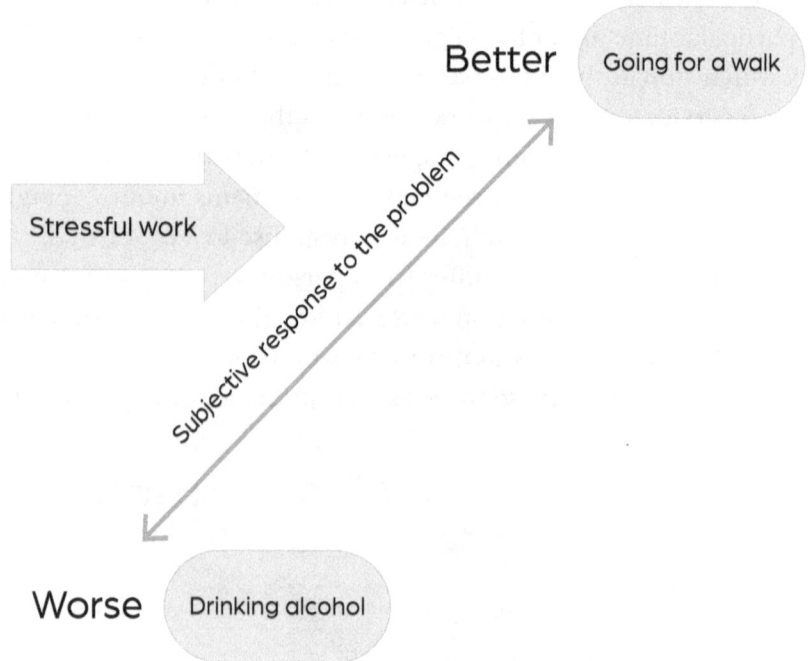

In our example, we have two common ways of coping with the problem of a stressful day at work. We placed them on the coping spectrum – the range of possible subjective responses to the problem. The spectrum goes from better to worse. Most would agree that going for a walk is a better way to cope with stress than drinking alcohol and so we place it higher on the spectrum than the use of alcohol.

We might also use the illustration to represent progress in learning how to cope better. Say, for example, at one time our friend typically had a few glasses of wine after work in order to relax, but after a while, she wanted to change this way of coping; so, she began to catch herself wanting to drink, and instead she'd decide to go for a walk; she intentionally made this decision again and again, and over time it became routine for her; she didn't have to decide between wine or walking every time – she just went for a walk, no longer thinking about it; as a result, she came to feel less stressed by work because she was now exercising rather than drinking; she came to find that engaging in a mild aerobic exercise was more effective than alcohol use. This person moved up the spectrum and came to cope better with the problem she experienced.

Notice too the important psychological change that occurred. Now that our friend is coping better, her actual experience of working is that it is less stressful than how it seemed when she was drinking wine in order to cope. The work remained the same, but she came to experience her work as less stressful because she was coping better.

Isn't this experience possible? Isn't it, in fact, common? We've all had the experience of coming to cope better with a problem and as a result, the problem becomes less problematic – even if the problem doesn't go away. Any parent recognizes that a crying baby in the middle of the night is easier to deal with if you've slept well the night before. If you're grounded, you typically respond to the baby better than when you've been up all the previous night and are therefore tired and stressed. The experience of the crying baby isn't different in each situation, the only thing that's different is you and how you're coping. When you cope better, your problems become more tolerable.

Think of the far-reaching ramifications of this simple fact about coping. By coping better, you can get to the point where problems become tolerable. Here we have a way to get better even if we can't entirely get rid of the problems that we face.

Now certainly, there are times when we try to fix our problems so that we then don't have to worry about how we're going to cope with them. We might even say that it should be the first thing to do. In our example, our friend should by all means try to resolve the problems at work so that it's less stressful. By doing so, she then doesn't have to worry about how she's going to cope with it or how she might cope better with it.

Of course, it's not always possible. We know that some jobs are just inherently stressful. We might make minimal progress in making them less stressful, but they're going to remain stressful overall. Examples such as police officers, firefighters, and junior high school teachers come to mind. The same is true with many problems in life. They are unfixable. While we might be able to minimize them to some degree, we ultimately have to put up with them. Is all hope lost then?

No, of course not! We get better by learning to cope more effectively with the unfixable problems of life. By coming to cope better, these unfixable problems become less problematic. We thereby free ourselves up to engage in life's activities and live well despite having certain problems. We do it all the time, every day of our lives.

Does this sound familiar? It should. Everything that we've said about coping with problems generally is true of coping with chronic pain. We might represent chronic pain and our subjective responses on the coping spectrum similarly to the other illustrations.

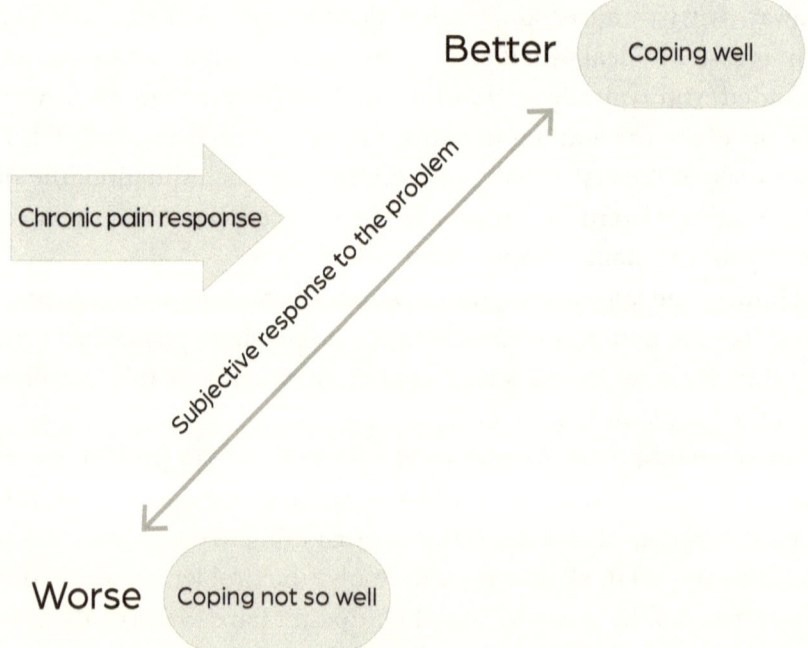

Suppose this illustration depicts a patient who has come to cope better with chronic pain.

At first, he wasn't coping well. There may have been many possible reasons for it: he had persistent insomnia and became irritable and depressed; maybe he's been a workaholic all his life and now, having had chronic pain for many years and being unable to work, he became prone to shame and self-criticism; maybe he lacked the self-confidence to engage in activities because of the pain activities cause and, as a result, he avoided going out and was largely home-bound. Whatever the case, he's not coping well and pain has taken over his life. Pain is literally intolerable. So, we place him at the low end of the coping spectrum to illustrate that he's not coping well. Notice too that we place his level of coping on the spectrum in an area that's lower than the pain. This location represents the fact that for him the pain is intolerable.

Now, suppose, he begins a CPRP in which he learns new ways to cope with pain. For instance, he works to resolve the secondary stressors (insomnia, depression, workaholism, fear-avoidance, among others). Over time, he comes to cope better. He sleeps better at night. He's no longer depressed. His self-esteem is no longer dependent on his productivity. He learned to pace himself and be satisfied when things are good enough. He became self-confident again and is out of the house, engaging in meaningful activities. In other words, he is coping well now. As a result, his pain has become less problematic. In fact, his pain, which was once intolerable, has become tolerable.

We depict his progress by placing him higher on the spectrum of coping. Notice too that we locate his coping responses higher than the pain to illustrate that the pain is now tolerable. He's on top of the pain and coping well.

There is great power in learning to cope better.

Here is where true hope lies. Getting better is possible and what it means for you to get better is that you change your subjective reactions to pain to the extent that pain becomes tolerable. You're already in the process of changing your locus of control from an external locus of control – the perspective that focuses on getting rid of pain by relying on others to do something to you – to an internal locus of control – the perspective that focuses on you by improving your subjective reactions to pain so that you're no longer alarmed or fearful or angry or depressed about being in pain; it becomes something that you put up with, but don't give a lot of attention to, like other unfixable problems in life.

Let's move on to more specific ways to cope better that we know are effective. We can differentiate these ways into two broad categories –resolving the secondary stressors that complicate pain and changing how you subjectively react to pain itself. For the remainder of this chapter, we'll focus on the former – increasing coping through overcoming the secondary stressors that occur when living with chronic pain. We'll focus on how to increase coping with pain itself in the next chapter.

Resolving the secondary stressors that complicate your pain

CPRPs focus on reducing the stressors that commonly occur when living with chronic pain because people cope better when they have fewer problems. It's like juggling. It's easier to juggle three balls than five or six or seven balls. So, the fewer the problems you have the better you'll cope with the pain that remains chronic.

So what are the common secondary problems that complicate chronic pain? We have previously listed them: insomnia, anxiety, depression, relationship problems, and work loss, among others. We discussed insomnia in the last chapter. In the remainder of this chapter, let's discuss the next three problems: overcoming anxiety, depression, and relationship problems. We'll save the loss of work for another chapter.

Overcoming anxiety

To my knowledge, there are no research studies showing what's the most common secondary problem that people with chronic pain have. Most people would likely say depression, but I'd put anxiety at the top of the list. It may surprise you.

Patients in CPRPs commonly don't think of themselves as anxious. They'll genuinely deny it when asked outright: "Do you have anxiety?" Nonetheless, they'll tend to answer affirmatively if asked, "Do you find yourself tense or restless?" or "Do people think you worry too much?" In fact, they often go on to report that their fretting and worry keep them up at night. They describe recurrent apprehensions about doing activities because of the pain involved or they speak of the dread they feel over whether to commit themselves to activities in the future, like family celebrations or holidays, as they may be unable to do it when the day arrives and so will face the conflict of having to let others down. As such, patients with chronic pain are often anxious, even if they don't ever think of themselves as "anxious," per se.

It makes sense that pain and anxiety tend to go together. In fact, it's as natural a pair as ketchup and mustard or peanut butter and jelly.

What is anxiety? There are many ways to answer the question. One way is to go back to our understanding of the nervous system. When anxious, we are *nervous* –literally. Our nervous system kicks into high gear. It becomes reactive. In other words, the nervous system goes into the stress, or fight-of-flight, response.

Recall what we learned in Chapter Four. The fight-or-flight response is our reaction to danger – our nervous system becomes reactive, leading to increased focus on the danger, increased energy, increased muscle tension, increased heart rate and blood pressure, increased reactivity in the gut, among other things. Because the nervous system also controls our emotional life, we come to feel either fear or anger or both. All this increased reactivity prepares and motivates us to respond to danger in order to survive – to either take it on (i.e., fight) or get out of there (i.e., flight). Once having successfully dealt with the danger, the nervous system returns to its normal relaxed state.

In Chapter Four, we saw that this stress response is also our response to pain. The function of pain is that it signals to us that something is wrong. It's a danger signal and the nervous system responds accordingly with increased reactivity. But unlike other dangers, chronic pain doesn't go away and so people with chronic pain never fully return back to a normal relaxed state.

So, you tend to persistently focus on the pain. You tend to experience chronic muscle tension and restlessness. You also tend to have recurrent fear and/or anger, which is to say, you have anxiety and irritability.

Another way to look at it is to review the difference between fear and anxiety. Have you ever thought about it? What's the difference between fear and anxiety? The notion of fight-or-flight comes in handy here too.

Fear is an emotion that we have in response to something dangerous. Physically, we feel the components of the fight-or-flight response that we listed above. Cognitively, we focus on the danger. Behaviorally, we are motivated to get away from the danger. Think, for example, how all these things would play out if we were walking late at night on a dark street and a suspicious group of individuals approached us.

Now, with anxiety, we have all the same reactions, but they occur in the absence of actual danger. We react to a danger that we think might happen. We feel anxious when, for instance, we worry about being unable to pay the bills. The worrying is our cognitive focus on the danger: being unable to pay the bills. Physically, we have increased tension, heart rate, blood pressure, and perspiration. Behaviorally, we are motivated to act. We have lots of energy, but there is nowhere to run.

There's nowhere to run because the danger isn't an actual thing that we can get away from. It's a potential danger that we are thinking might happen. As such, we're all tensed up with nowhere to go. So, we're fidgety and can't sit still.

It's what happens when living with chronic pain, right? The nervous system reacts to pain as the danger signal it is and so the nervous system prepares us to take action, but there's no action to take. You are all tensed up with nowhere to go. You can't get away from the pain. Yet, you can't just stop your nervous system from reacting. You're stuck in fight-or-flight, which, at the end of the day, is simply anxiety.

Here we see how chronic pain naturally leads to anxiety. They go hand in hand.

Patients in a CPRP tend to ask, at this point, what can we do about it? Thankfully, there's a lot you can do about it.

Before discussing them, let's make a quick comment. Our goal in this section is to provide concrete ways to reduce the garden-variety anxiety you have when living with chronic pain. This type of anxiety wouldn't necessarily constitute an anxiety disorder diagnosis, such as panic disorder and the like. In other words, you probably have anxiety like we described above and you should focus on reducing it because it'll help you to cope better with chronic pain, but the fact that you may have this level of anxiety doesn't necessarily mean you could be diagnosed with an anxiety disorder. Now having said that, sometimes people with chronic pain also have an actual anxiety disorder and so we'll end this section with some thoughts on how to get further help if you do.

Next steps. The first thing to do is to accept that chronic pain tends to make you anxious. Hopefully, the above discussion helps you see how it occurs. Once you accept that it's happening, you can begin to do something about it.

It's helpful here to recognize that you're already reducing your pain-related anxiety. How? Well, by this far into your program, you should already be engaging in a daily relaxation therapy and some type of regular mild aerobic exercise. As we've discussed, these therapies are helpful because they down-regulate your overly reactive nervous system. The emotional correlation to an up-regulated nervous system is anxiety and irritability. With regular relaxation and mild aerobic exercise, you are working to reduce anxiety (and pain, of course) by intervening at the level of your nervous system.

Moreover, you should already be intervening at the behavioral level of your pain and anxiety mix. How? You are committed to stopping pain talk and pain behaviors – the public expressions of being in pain. You are attempting to catch yourself as you get up from the chair, for instance, with a groan, grimace and grab at the site of pain.

It's important because, with the groan, grimace, and grab, you're reacting to pain with alarm. Your reaction reinforces the perspective that your pain is really a dangerous thing to which you should be reacting in startling ways – the groan, grimace, and grab. It's also emotionally upsetting. Almost always when reacting in these ways, patients comment on how bad it is. It also broadcasts this sense of alarm to others around you and they too get upset and fly into rescue mode. It's like flashing the red-alert sign and ringing the alarm bells and everyone is getting tensed up with nowhere to go.

Instead, you've been attempting to observe yourself, catch yourself in these alarming reactions, and refrain from engaging in them. In other words, you are practicing having pain while at the same time remaining grounded, which is to say, not anxious.

Let's now review more ways to reduce anxiety. These ways attempt to change the emotional experience of anxiety and the thinking that goes along with anxiety.

Changing your emotional experiences. In ancient Greece, before the time of the great philosophers like Socrates, Plato, and Aristotle, there stood a temple in a town called Delphi. Inscribed on the temple wall were the simple words: *Know thyself.* Ever since, great thinkers, writers, and healthcare providers keep coming back to this simple truth.

The simple truth is that something important happens when you start paying attention to yourself and your surroundings. You slow down. You become more reflective and deliberative. And as a result, you change your perspective on things.

It takes the pressure off you when you see that there are more ways than one to understand an issue. So often, we get upset when it seems we have to choose between a limited set of bad options, as if it's either this way or that way. When you step out of the moment and reflect on how you are feeling, it takes you out of the automatic reactions that occur in response to daily events, and provides you with emotional breathing room, as it were. As a consequence, you settle down. Let's look at how to do this intentionally.

One of the most influential thinkers who took up this simple truth in recent times was a Viennese neurologist in the late 19th century who began to treat disorders of the nervous system by establishing a trusting relationship with his patients and talking to them about their problems. His name was Sigmund Freud and he was one of the first healthcare providers to set out a method for treating patients psychologically, as opposed to medically. Since his time, it's been known that one of the most effective components of all psychological therapies is to show patients how to pay attention to their thoughts and feelings, and their reactions to events. Borrowing from the tradition Freud started, we have called it developing an *observational self* in this book.

One way to develop the ability to step out of any given moment and reflect on how you're reacting is to practice the ability to recognize your feelings. It's a difficult skill to develop, even though most people initially think it's easy. "Who doesn't know what they're feeling?" one might ask. The truth is that we hardly ever take the time to slow down and reflect on how we're thinking or feeling about the events of our lives. In the course of our day, we go about our business routinely doing this and that, reacting to this and that, and making split-second decisions, without ever giving it much thought. That is to say, we often don't know what it is we're feeling.

When directly asked, most times we say something like, 'Well, I feel good' or 'I feel bad.' It's a common, everyday statement. Now, if you stop and think about it, you might notice that 'good' and 'bad' aren't feelings. Rather, they are judgments about the value of something, whether we like it or not, whether it has worth or importance or not. The use of 'good' or 'bad' categorizes our feelings into two kinds, but they don't allow us to know what we're really feeling. When we say, "I feel good (or bad)," we are really saying, "I feel something – don't actually know what – but I like (or don't like) it."

Indeed, often, we can be upset and not fully know why or even how. We're all tensed up with nowhere to go. We start to do one thing, get reminded of another, start that one, and then get distracted and start doing a third thing, without ever getting any one of them completed. Maybe, we find ourselves eating things we shouldn't and don't ever stop to reflect that we aren't really hungry, but rather worried. Or we find ourselves yelling at the kids, without ever reflecting that it's not really them, it's us; we're actually tense and restless, and so are finding that every little thing bugs us more than it should.

In the past, psychologists used the word 'unconscious' to describe such feelings and reactions, but this word seems to make it more mysterious than it is. We now use the word 'automatic' to describe these types of feelings and reactions. It's a helpful word to use because it gets at the notion that we react to things without much thought about it. We do them without really intending to do them. They are automatic.

You can begin to get a handle on your anxiety (or any distressing emotion for that matter) by simply identifying the feeling you have. By recognizing the anxiety for what it is, you change the tone of the emotional experience. It stops the subtle sense of helplessness that occurs when it feels like things are getting away from you and you don't know why. You recognize that you're not hungry, you're just eating because you're worried. By paying attention, you realize that it's not really the kids who are upsetting you, it's you who is upset. Having an accurate understanding of your feelings changes the emotional experience for the better because you can then take ownership of your reactions. As a result, you say, something like, "I'm sorry. I'm not angry with you. I'm just short-fused because I'm anxious about…" By owning it, you settle everyone down.

Once you're able to identify your feelings and own them, you can take a moment to decide what to do about them. You might, for example, choose to engage in diaphragmatic breathing or you might go for a walk or talk about your anxieties with friends or loved ones. These practices further help you to see that there are different perspectives that you might take.

By observing your feelings, identifying them, and deciding what to do about them, you also change the emotional pressure you feel to act when having anxiety. When anxious, we feel pressure to do something. We are tense and restless. We are in some degree of fight-or-flight with nowhere to go. However, when you recognize that you're anxious, you take the pressure off. You don't have to fly by the seat of your pants. You can slow down and deliberate on how to react.

In other words, you step out of the moment and observe yourself. From your observational self, you have the breathing room to begin practicing a different reaction – one that is hopefully healthier and more effective than your usual automatic response.

To sum up, learning to recognize your feelings is a way to develop an observational self that allows you to step out of any given moment and reflect on how you're reacting and choose a healthier and more effective way to react. You thereby change the actual emotional experience of anxiety (or any other distressing emotion).

This is what good coping looks like. You change your subjective reaction by fostering the ability to know yourself – stepping out of your automatic responses and observing them, reflecting on them, and making an intentional choice of how to respond.

Obviously, changing your emotional experiences through self-observation takes practice. You have to remember to practice it. I encourage patients to use things that help them to remember. Sticky notes can be used for this purpose. Take some sticky notes and write 'Stop, breathe, identify feeling' on them. Place one on the bathroom mirror, one on the refrigerator, and one on the door out to the garage. They'll prompt you to remember to stop for a moment, take a deep diaphragmatic breath, and reflect on what you're thinking and feeling. Another trick is to have a small item that you keep in your front pocket and its only purpose is to trigger you to stop, breathe, and identify what you're feeling whenever you touch it. It might be a smooth stone or a medallion or some old lucky charm that's been hiding out in a junk drawer. Keep it in your front pocket and every time you touch it, accidentally or otherwise, take a moment to diaphragmatically breathe and reflect on how you are feeling right then and there. In these ways, you practice observing yourself, which you use to change how you feel and how you're reacting to the events of life. As you practice, it gets easier and easier and becomes a new healthy habit.

Talking about your feelings helps. Now that you're practicing to recognize your feelings, find a few confidants with whom you can share them. Obviously, your psychologist and other CPRP providers are key figures here. The other patients in your CPRP are important too. However, you might have other confidants as well, such as your spouse, a friend, a close relative, or the leader of your religious community. It's important to have people in your life in whom to confide because sharing your feelings is healthy.

The old saying that 'two heads are better than one' is typically true when it comes to overcoming problems. It's also true for overcoming anxiety. When we talk about our feelings with others, we tend to have insights we might not have had alone. We gain perspective. Oftentimes, it becomes clear how to move forward and resolve the anxiety.

When we share our feelings, we create intimacy in our relationships. We know that we aren't alone and that people care. We know we have another person in the world who will bear witness to our trials and support our attempts to resolve them. Such intimacy is reassuring and it reduces anxiety even further.

We also know that expressing feelings can lead to a host of health improvements. Over a few decades, researchers at the University of Texas led by James Pennebaker, a psychologist, have found that expressing your feelings is healthy across a number of domains (Pennebaker, 1997; Pennebaker & Chung, 2011). In a series of experiments, they found that people who verbally (or in writing, such as in a journal) express their distressing feelings come to have less anxiety and feel like they can move on from problems they experience. Pennebaker and colleagues have also found that people who express or share their feelings seek healthcare less often and have higher immune system functioning. Sharing your feelings also lowers the reactivity of your nervous system, as measured by such things as heart rate and blood pressure. As we know, by lowering nervous system reactivity, we become less anxious.

It's important then that you share your feelings with those who you trust. Coupled with recognizing your feelings, it's an effective way to overcome anxiety.

Changing your anxious thinking. In the last two sections, we've discussed the emotional experience of anxiety – the tension, nervousness, apprehension, and dread. We've also discussed the physical side of anxiety – the increased energy, muscle tension, heart rate, perspiration, upset stomach, and the like. We've also mentioned the behavioral aspects to anxiety – being fidgety, restless, and unable to sit still. Let's now talk about the cognitive aspects of anxiety – the thinking that goes along with anxiety.

As we've discussed, one of the things that happens in the fight-or-flight response is that we become cognitively focused on the danger to which we're reacting. We noted that attention becomes focused on the danger and subsequently we typically don't have random distracting thoughts. In Chapter Four, we used the example of slamming on the brakes of a vehicle to keep from hitting a child who runs into the road. We mentioned that, in the immediacy of such a situation, we wouldn't have distracted thoughts like, whether we have the right ingredients for tonight's dinner. Rather, our thoughts and attention become focused on braking and missing the child.

A similar cognitive focus happens when anxious, though with an important difference. We're in fight-or-flight, but unable to fight or flee because the danger to which we're reacting is not an actual danger, but one that might happen. That is to say, we are thinking about a possible bad thing happening. We call it worry.

Worry is the cognitive focus of fight-or-flight when something bad might happen, as opposed to something that's actually happening. Our automatic reactions, however, don't know the difference. We get just as revved up when anticipating something bad happening as we do when something bad is actually happening.

Psychologists have noticed that we all tend to worry in some similar ways. We call them *automatic negative thoughts* to refer to the fact that they occur without much intention. We have them without wanting them to occur (i.e. they're automatic). They are also always about bad things happening (i.e., they're negative). We all tend to have automatic negative thoughts but when we're anxious we tend to have them a lot. Let's review two common types of such thoughts.

The first is what we call *catastrophization*. We catastrophize when we automatically think of the worst-case scenario and subsequently think that it's going to happen. It has two aspects: thinking about the worst-case scenario and overestimating the likelihood of it occurring. Catastrophizations often start with the words "What if…" We fill in the blank by thinking that something terribly bad, or catastrophic, might happen. We subsequently begin to get physically and emotionally worked up as if it is inevitably bound to happen. As such, we overestimate the likelihood that it will occur.

In everyday language, we tend to refer to catastrophizing with such phrases as "making a mountain out of a molehill" or "crossing a bridge before you get to it."

Chronic pain patients tend to catastrophize in many ways. Some common ones are the belief that they're inevitably going to get worse or more disabled; or they think of the worst level of pain they ever had in the past and anticipate that they'll have that level again when doing everyday things, tending to forget about the more common occurrences when they do things with mild to moderate pain levels.

Such thinking reflects anxiety, but it also promotes it. When you think of your condition in drastic, inevitably deteriorating ways, the future looks pretty bleak. Once convinced of a bleak future, you feel pretty vulnerable to things that can go wrong. Pain seems always just around the corner and so activities are to be dreaded and avoided. Such persistent dread saps your self-confidence, leaving you more vulnerable and anxious. Catastrophization is thus both a product of anxiety and a catalyst for more anxiety.

A second type of anxious thinking is *all-or-nothing thinking*. It occurs when we think of something as having to be either this way or that way with no inbetween. In such situations, we fail to notice the complexities of events and so the stakes get high. We feel pressure because we're stuck between a rock and a hard place.

Chronic pain patients can tend to engage in all-or-nothing thinking. It's quite common for patients to tell me that on a good day, they clean their entire house all at once because they let it go for so long. It's like they have only two options: either do it all at once or not at all. Oftentimes, patients think that they either have to go back to work in exactly the way they used to do or they are totally and permanently disabled. Such thinking reflects a nervous system in persistent vigilance, but it is also anxiety provoking. The stakes are high if you have only two choices, both of which are bad.

To change your anxious thinking, we follow the same route we have for changing anxious feelings. First, try to catch yourself having such thoughts. Typically, when we catastrophize or engage in all-or-nothing thinking, it never occurs to us that such thoughts are untrue or that we could see things differently. However, having begun to foster an observational self, you might begin to notice when you're doing it.

It also helps to label these thoughts for what they are – catastrophizations and all-or-nothing thinking. It puts them in a light that begins to doubt their accuracy – that they don't really represent the situation at hand. For example, if I can see that my thinking is really catastrophizing, then it naturally leads to entertaining the thought that maybe... just maybe... the situation isn't as drastically bad as I initially thought it to be. Similarly, if I can come to see and label my thinking as an example of all-or-nothing thinking, then I can begin to entertain the possibility that maybe... just maybe... there are more options available to me besides the perceived no-win situation. By observing and identifying such thoughts as specific automatic negative thoughts, you begin to change your perspective.

Once you've recognized that you're doing it, try to challenge the accuracy of your automatic negative thoughts. Let's take catastrophizations. How true is it that the worst-case scenario is bound to happen? Remember that catastrophizations have two characteristics – thinking of the worst-case scenario and overestimating the likelihood that it'll happen. Now, you might recognize that, usually, worst-case scenarios, while possible, are highly unlikely. Suppose you just 'know' that you're inevitably going to end up in a wheelchair because of low back pain. Consider how common low back pain is in the general population and ask yourself how often does paralysis really occur because of back pain? Do you know anyone who became wheelchair-bound? Probably not. If, by chance, you do know someone who became wheelchair-bound because of low back pain, the person either had some other condition that made them paralyzed (as low back pain doesn't typically cause paralysis) or the person became wheel-chair bound because of getting out of shape and becoming too weak to stand or walk for any length of time – not a true paralysis. Notice that this worst-case scenario is completely preventable through your exercise regimen. So, once you identify that the thought is a catastrophization, you challenge it by considering the true likelihood of its occurrence. Upon further reflection, you come to realize that worst-case scenarios rarely, if ever, happen.

To overcome all-or-nothing thinking, you do the same process. You observe the thought and recognize to yourself that you're engaged in all-or-nothing thinking. After identifying it for what it is, you challenge it by paying attention to the complexities of the situation. Who says you must let your house go for days on end and then clean it in its entirety the moment you have a little less pain? Who made that rule? And is it really a good pain management strategy to bounce back and forth from nothing to everything? It's perfectly acceptable – and preferable! – to practice pacing yourself.

What you're trying to do in changing your anxious thinking is to make your responses to situations less automatic and more thoughtful or intentional. When engaged in catastrophizing or all-or-nothing thinking, it seems so accurate to what's really going on that we never give it much thought. We're simply anxious and perceive the situation in a drastic, either-or way, which both reflects our anxiety at the time and provokes it still further. By observing these thoughts and challenging them, we begin to question their apparent accuracy and intentionally reflect on different ways to see the situation. It gives us breathing room to consider a different way to approach the situation and it takes the pressure off. It leads to less anxiety.

Like everything else in this book, it takes practice to catch yourself in automatic negative thoughts and challenge them. When you see your sticky notes or feel your stone or medallion in your pocket, stop for a moment, take a deep breath, and consider what you're feeling and what you're thinking. See if you're engaged in catastrophizing or all-or-nothing thinking. Challenge its accuracy and talk about them with your psychologist and other providers, the patients in your CPRP, and your trusted loved ones.

What to do if you have an actual anxiety disorder. We've been discussing how to overcome the run-of-the-mill anxiety that comes with chronic pain, not how to treat an actual diagnosable anxiety disorder like panic disorder or post-traumatic stress disorder. We should mention a few pointers for those who do in fact have (or think they might have) such a disorder. After all, it's common that chronic pain patients also have anxiety disorders.

You should discuss your concerns about having an anxiety disorder with your CPRP providers. They should be able to diagnose it if you do and they should also be able to recommend and offer a course of treatment.

The treatment recommendations typically include psychotherapy. Among mental healthcare experts, psychotherapy is recognized as the most effective treatment for anxiety disorders (Heuzenroeder, et al., 2004; Mitte, 2005; Otto, Smits, & Reese, 2005). Psychotherapy can assist you in curing an anxiety disorder. Now, it doesn't lead to a cure for everyone and, even for those who can resolve their anxiety disorder, they'll still occasionally have anxiety, as some degree of anxiety comes with life. But, by and large, people can get to the point where the level and frequency of anxiety no longer reaches the point that they'd meet the criteria for an anxiety disorder diagnosis.

CPRP providers also commonly recommend taking an antidepressant medication. Patients are often taken aback by the recommendation, particularly if they don't see themselves as depressed. However, among medications, antidepressants are the most effective medication to take for anxiety (Nutt, 2005). Indeed, in the short term, taking an antidepressant medication is largely as effective as psychotherapy. However, over the long term, this effectiveness diminishes. Moreover, the original high levels of anxiety typically return once patients discontinue the medication, if they haven't been in psychotherapy and have learned how to control and prevent their anxiety. This finding is what makes psychotherapy more effective than just the medication alone – patients don't lose their knowledge of how to control and prevent anxiety once psychotherapy is discontinued (Gould, Otto, Pollack & Yap, 1997).

CPRP providers typically recommend against taking certain anti-anxiety medications (or recommend that you taper these types of medication if you're already taking one). These recommendations may also be surprising. The type of anti-anxiety medications in question are sedatives, called benzodiazepines. Common forms are diazepam, alprazolam, clonazepam, or lorazepam. When used on a brief basis to help you cope with a big event that makes you anxious, there may be nothing necessarily bad about it. So, for example, sometimes patients with a fear of flying might take one prior to their departure and return flights. When used in this brief manner, they are largely considered safe. However, there are problems associated with these medications when taken on a regular basis.

It's long been known that they produce rebound anxiety (Chouinard 2004; Kales, et al., 1983; Power, et al., 1985; Rynn & Brawman-Mintzer, 2004). What happens is that the sedative reduces your anxiety while it's in your system, but once it wears off, your anxiety returns to higher levels than what it was before taking the medication. Patients tend to respond to the increased anxiety with more use of the sedative, which in turn leads to more rebound anxiety. As such, they can become very difficult to stop taking.

On top of it all, they are also addictive. The medications do more than just reduce anxiety when in your system. They produce euphoria. People can come to like this feeling too much and become classically addicted. So, CPRP providers tend to recommend against the use of these medications.

Before making any medication changes, you should always talk to the providers who are prescribing them. They know you and your particular conditions the best. There are also significant health issues at stake when tapering medications, particularly benzodiazepines, and it needs to be done correctly or you can put your health in jeopardy.

Overcoming anxiety leads to improved coping with pain. Everything in life is harder to deal with when anxious. You're alarmed and your body and behavior, your thoughts and feelings, reflect it. Anxiety colors your perceptions. Difficult-to-cross bridges need to be anticipated and crossed before even getting to them. Molehills can seem like mountains. Any problems, not just the small stuff, seem insurmountable.

Getting grounded, though, helps. You think clearer and you tend to see problems more accurately. You can reality-check your catastrophizations and can think of alternatives to the either-or options that initially come to mind. The problems of life become less alarming and you cope better with them.

Notice, then, what happens. You move up the spectrum of coping. By overcoming anxiety, everything – including chronic pain – becomes less problematic. Remaining grounded helps to make problems easier to deal with. It's one of the ways that you can make tolerable what was once intolerable.

Overcoming depression

Depression is common with chronic pain. There are many reasons for it. Chronic pain and anxiety are depressing. Loss of work and loss of your role in the family or community are blows to your self-esteem and can make the future seem hopeless. Stressed relationships with your spouse and family lead to conflict and resentment, which are also depressing. We could go on, of course.

Depression makes pain harder to cope with. It makes everything harder to cope with. If we represented it in our coping spectrum illustration, the onset of depression can lead you to move down the coping spectrum. Depression can be one of the many secondary factors, which go into making pain intolerable. However, overcoming depression makes pain more tolerable. So, let's review how to overcome it.

We should review a caveat. Depression could have its own self-help manual. It would lead us too far astray to review everything you need to know to treat depression per se. In this section, we'll review overcoming depression as it relates to living with chronic pain. Pursuing these recommendations may be sufficient for the typical mild depression that comes with chronic pain. However, if you're moderately or severely depressed, or if you were depressed before you developed pain, you should go beyond what's recommended in this book. Talk to your CPRP providers or obtain care with a psychologist who'll be able to help you and direct your care.

The first thing to do is to recognize all the antidepressant activities that you're doing in your CPRP. You've accepted the chronicity of your pain and have begun to empower yourself to self-manage it as the way to get better. No longer looking for a cure that never comes, you've let go of false hope and have come to have a true hope. You've also begun a regular aerobic exercise and daily relaxation therapy, both of which are down-regulating your nervous system. You're focused on improving your sleep. As such, you may have less fatigue and irritability. You're also refraining from pain talk and pain behaviors. As you become more adept at controlling your alarming reactions to pain, you become less somatically focused and your relationships may improve as a result.

You've also begun to work on reducing anxiety through developing an observational self, recognizing and talking about your feelings, and challenging your automatic negative thoughts.

All of these healthy changes aid to overcome depression. In fact, we might assert that by doing them you get at the cause of the common depression that occurs with chronic pain. When the nervous system is up-regulated, and pain has become chronic through the process of central sensitization, it leads to chronic anxiety and other stressors which, over time, are physically and emotionally exhausting, or depressing. Everything you've learned so far in your CPRP is leading to a reversal of this overall condition.

Let's discuss a few interventions that are geared to overcome depression per se.

More automatic negative thoughts. In the previous section, we reviewed two kinds of automatic negative thoughts, catastrophizations, and all-or-nothing thinking. They aren't, however, the only types of automatic negative thoughts that people have.

We all make critical judgments of ourselves. How often do you say to yourself, "Oh, that was stupid" or "that sounded dumb…" when interacting with others. This kind of thought flits by in the course of our everyday lives and we hardly ever notice them. However, we do tend to believe them.

We call these types of thoughts our *inner critic*. It's like we have an inner critic who delivers a running commentary on our behavior in the course of our daily lives. We might hardly ever notice it because of its almost life-long familiarity. We certainly never question its accuracy. Its critical judgments, we typically assume, are true.

Now, depression can be considered from various angles, but one way to think about what happens when you become depressed is that you not only believe your inner critic, but you personalize it. Everyone, whether depressed or not, might tend to think, for example, that something we said was stupid on occasion. When depressed, though, we think that we really are stupid for saying it. Notice the difference. In the first case, it's the behavior that you think is stupid. In the second, it's you who are stupid. Your belief in the accuracy of your inner criticisms crosses a line from what you did to who you really are. You just "know" that you're bad – not just your behavior in that one instance.

It is, of course, the source of the low self-esteem of depression. It naturally leads to the recurrent sense that you don't deserve things to go well.

Once self-esteem is low, you have ample occasion for more inner criticisms. Almost anything you might do is open for negative judgment –food for the fodder. It's a common vicious cycle that leads to depression.

Just as with catastrophizations and all-or-nothing thinking, you can get a handle on the automatic negative judgments by catching yourself having them, challenging their accuracy, and practicing maintaining the perspective that they are untrue. We say in raising a child, "criticize the behavior, not the child." Why? Well, we want the child to see the misbehavior as bad but not themselves as bad. We can all readily see this principle get broken when watching parents or other adults do it to children. We readily intervene and reassure the child that they're okay – it's just their misbehavior that's not okay. Right? It's easily seen and done when witnessing it happen to a child. So, why is it so hard to see when we do it to ourselves? The depressed person breaks this principle all the time and never gives it much thought.

However, you can start paying attention to when you do it. You catch yourself criticizing yourself, label it for what it is, and consider whether you're really that bad. Say you make a poorly timed comment at a party and your inner critic starts letting you have it. This time, though, you catch yourself and try to see your comment more accurately. Your inner criticism is usually worse than the actual deed that was done. Maybe, you talk with a friend to see if what you said was as bad as your inner critic thinks it is. By reality-checking your inner critic in these ways, you challenge its accuracy and come to see that you don't have to believe the negative judgment of yourself. You then repeat this process whenever you can catch your inner critic. With time, it has less control over how you think of yourself and you become less depressed.

Another common type of automatic negative thinking is *I-can't-thinking.* I-can't-thinking occurs when, just as it sounds, you tell yourself that you can't do things, which, upon closer inspection, you might still be able to do. Now, of course, there are things that we really can't do, like jumping to the moon, and if you were to tell yourself "I can't jump to the moon," you aren't engaged in this type of automatic negative thought. Rather, I-can't-thinking occurs when you think you can't do something, which you likely can do. You might be familiar with the notion of I-can't-thinking, but have used a different, more common phrase for it – psyching yourself out. We're familiar with the everyday experience of people who psych themselves out, believing that they can't do something as they get up to do it, never recognizing that they might reasonably be able to do what it is they're trying to do – if only they stopped their I-can't-thinking.

Let's take an example. Depressed chronic pain patients often say, without much reflection, something like, "Oh, I can't go to the party." They say it as matter-of-fact and go on in the conversation as if the statement is simply and obviously true. If asked why they can't go, they typically respond with statements that they can't because of the pain. This thought naturally leads to feeling down about their situation in life. But, how true is it that they can't go? The word "can't" means to be unable to do something or that something is impossible to do. It's on the order of something like a blind person who can't see or a paralyzed person who can't walk. Does pain rise to that level? Might it be true that when a depressed chronic pain patient says, "I can't go to the party," she is engaged in I-can't-thinking because it isn't really true that she's unable to go or that it's impossible to go?

Whether you're depressed or in pain or both, you can still move your arms and legs and get to a party.

Now, of course, the individual in question might not want to go or may have to get there differently than in the past or may want to stay for only a period of time – these statements may very well be true. But, it isn't true that she is unable to attend a party. Thinking and saying, "I can't go to the party," is an example of I-can't-thinking.

Maybe you engage in I-can't-thinking too? Patients commonly use the word "can't" in relation to the fact that they aren't working or pursuing recreational activities, doing household chores, or dressing or bathing themselves. Patients think that they "just can't" do these activities and they treat the thought as if it's matter-of-factly true because they're too depressed or have too much pain or both.

Now, at this point, many patients get upset with me when I talk like this.

They react that I just don't get it. If I understood the pain they have, they say, then I'd know that the I-can't-thinking is true – that it's not an example of an automatic negative thought, but rather an accurate description of their abilities.

It's a sensitive issue.

As I do with my patients, I would ask that you simply consider the notion of I-can't-thinking as a type of automatic negative thinking. There is a lot at stake. I-can't-thinking is one of the causes of depression in chronic pain patients and learning how to change it can be one of the ways you overcome depression.

I-can't-thinking leads to depression because of the loss of activities with which it's associated. Once you start to believe that you can't do things that others take for granted, such as working, household chores, social activities, and the like, a whole host of distressing feelings can follow. You start to feel helpless. You start to feel dependent on others, which in turn leads to self-criticism and low self-esteem. You begin to feel more and more vulnerable – if today, you can't work or do yard work, it seems just a matter of time before you can't do other things. You might even find yourself jealous of others who are out doing things, which you wish you could still do. It's a bad mix of feelings to have. You feel helpless, vulnerable, dependent, and angry with yourself. If it goes on for too long, it's almost inevitable that you'll lose your motivation for the activities of life. In other words, it all equals depression. There's almost a logic to it.

So, before you dismiss this discussion because of the sensitivity it generates, consider that it may be to your benefit to give this notion of I-can't-thinking a second look. The question then becomes how do you start getting a handle on it and change this type of automatic negative thinking given the pain?

Just as we've discussed with other types of automatic negative thoughts, you repetitively try to observe yourself engaged in such thinking, label it for what it is, and challenge how accurate it is to the reality of the situation.

Suppose you hear yourself saying, "I can't" to someone. Consider for a moment, what you just did. Perhaps, you say to yourself, "Oh, there I go again." Subsequently, you reflect, how true is it? Is it really impossible to do? Maybe, there are times when you could do the activity in question. Maybe, you'd have to do it differently than you have in the past, but nonetheless, you could still do it. For instance, you do it for less time than you've done in the past or you do it with the support of others. Recall that most situations don't rise to the level of impossibility. At the very least, it would be helpful to begin to acknowledge and practice saying to yourself that you don't want to do it because it will lead to too much pain, but also acknowledging that you could do it if it was worth it to you. It's important to acknowledge these things as it keeps you in control – you are the decision maker, not the pain.

Once having identified the automatic thought, challenged it, and come to see that it isn't necessarily true, you repeat this process over and over again. Again, it's like breaking a habit and the habit is a particular type of thinking. Over time, you get better at overcoming your automatic negative thoughts, and you begin to put yourself out there, doing more things, seeing that they're possible to do – albeit differently than you used to do them. You subsequently start to gain confidence.

You feel more in control of your day-to-day life. In other words, you start to feel empowered. Life seems a little brighter, more full of possibilities. You start to feel hopeful. You start to overcome depression.

Engage in pleasurable activities. Chronic pain and depression can get you in a rut. It's literally no fun. In fact, a symptom of depression is reduced interest in doing activities that you once found enjoyable. When depressed, you tend to tell your friends and family, "Ah, go without me... I'll just stay home." After a while, a life without pleasure is itself depressing. It's one of the many vicious cycles of chronic pain and depression.

One way to break the cycle is to make the intentional commitment to start doing fun activities, even if you initially don't feel like doing them. When a friend asks you to do something, make the effort to do it. Don't wait until you feel like doing it. Trust that by getting yourself out there, you'll eventually come to want to do these things again. You might surprise yourself and find that you enjoy it.

Patients at this point often counter by stating, "But I can't do what I used to do." Such statements bring us back to our previous discussion: you'll have to be working on your I-can't-thinking, catching yourself, labeling it, challenging how accurate it is to the situation, and coming up with a way to do the activity, even if you have done it differently than in the past. Automatic thoughts fly by without much reflection and seem so accurate that they're an instantaneous deal-killer. You have to identify and challenge them.

So, repetitively make the decision to do an activity and be open to how you might do it, rather than automatically shutting it down with "I can't." By doing so, you succeed in getting out of the house and bringing some pleasure and purpose back to life. In other words, it's a way to overcome depression.

Psychotherapy. Psychotherapy is a therapeutic activity in which you develop a trusting relationship with a healthcare provider and talk about your problems, identify their causes, develop the ability to observe them occurring in the moment and change how you respond to them in order to resolve them in some meaningful way.

People tend to associate psychotherapy with mental health problems. However, healthcare providers use and always have used, psychotherapy for health problems too. For instance, Freud, who initially developed psychotherapy as a treatment, was a neurologist who treated patients with what we'd now consider neurological conditions. Even today, psychotherapy is used, in combination with other therapies, for conditions as diverse as type II diabetes, heart disease, chronic gastrointestinal conditions, and cancer. So, it isn't so surprising that it is used for chronic pain.

Psychotherapy is usually done on an individual basis or in a group with other patients. As discussed in the introduction to this book, CPRPs employ both types of psychotherapy. Group psychotherapy is structured with a different topic each day, ranging from depression, anxiety, stress management, insomnia, and relationship problems. Individual psychotherapy in most programs is less structured, where you can explore and work on issues that are specific to you and your history.

Mental health experts agree that psychotherapy is apt to be the most effective treatment for depression (Spielman, Berman, Usitalo, 2011). In recent years, despite its effectiveness, psychotherapy has fallen out of public view as a treatment for depression, overshadowed by antidepressant medications. Many attribute this change in societal views to marketing strategies of the pharmaceutical industry, among other organizations (cf. Blumner & Marcus, 2009; Lacasse, 2005). Despite this change in views, the research is consistent: psychotherapy is as effective as antidepressants in the short-term and more effective in the long term (Antonuccio & Danton, 1995; DeRubeis, Gelfand, Tang, & Simons, 1999; Dobson, et al., 2008, Hollon, Stewart, Strunk, 2006; Hollon, et al., 2005).

The benefits of antidepressant medications tend to go away once you stop taking them, but the benefits of psychotherapy remain long after you stop the psychotherapy. In fact, there's significant evidence that, at least among some forms of psychotherapy, you continue to get better even after you stop the therapy (Shedler, 2010). It's probably because in psychotherapy you learn the skills to keep from getting depressed and, like any other skill, the more you practice them the better you get at them. However you slice it, psychotherapy is helpful in overcoming depression.

If you aren't currently participating in a CPRP and are experiencing depression, it's important that you begin psychotherapy with a psychologist who has knowledge and experience in chronic pain rehabilitation. At various times in this book, we've discussed the importance of having an expert healthcare provider with whom you can establish a trusting relationship and with whom you can work on self-managing pain through lifestyle changes and coping. To do both, you must work on the secondary problems that occur because of chronic pain. Depression is one of the most common of these secondary problems. So, to be successful in self-managing pain, you need to work on overcoming depression and psychotherapy is an effective way of doing it.

Antidepressant medications. You should also discuss with your CPRP providers the possible use of antidepressant medication. Antidepressants are effective in reducing depression (Arroll, et al., 2005; Williams, et al., 2000). It's important to acknowledge, though, that they don't cure depression. Patients sometimes complain that they're still depressed, even though they're on an antidepressant. However, the medications just aren't that effective (Fournier, et al., 2010; Kirsch et al., 2008; Matthew & Charney, 2009; Moncrieff & Kirsch, 2005). Once in a while, you run across a person who feels dramatically better when taking an antidepressant, but most people don't have that level of response. The commercials on television are misleading in this way.

Antidepressant medications are, however, often worth taking. Patients often feel brighter; they report that they tolerate the frustrations of life better and don't get irritated or tearful so easily. These improvements are worth having and antidepressants can help.

Antidepressant medications have also long been known to reduce pain because of their effect on the central nervous system (Hauser, Bernardy, Uceyler, & Sommer, 2009; Salerno, Browning, & Jackson, 2002; Saarto & Wiffen, 2007). CPRP providers thus use antidepressants to help patients cope better with pain, by being less depressed, and to actually reduce pain itself. Use of an antidepressant is a 2-for-1 deal.

Overcoming depression leads to improved coping with pain. Everything in life is harder to handle when depressed. It takes everything down a few notches. Fun things are no longer fun. Humorous things are no longer funny. The normal stressors of life that you generally would take in stride are now irritating and troubling. The big problems that are usually hard to manage are now overwhelming. It can get hard to even go on.

When you overcome depression, however, your perceptions realign themselves upward. Fun things are pleasurable again and jokes are funny again. Normal stressors return to being nuisances and you get back to work on the big problems of life.

Notice what happens. Nothing about life changes. Rather, you change. You move up the coping spectrum. Improving your mood makes life brighter. It's easier to deal with things. Indeed, you cope better with everything – including chronic pain. Overcoming depression is thus one of the ways that you make tolerable what was once intolerable.

Overcoming relationship problems

Before ending this chapter, we need to discuss another common stressor that results from living with chronic pain. It's relationship problems. Chronic pain is not only stressful for you, it's also stressful for your loved ones. They feel bad for you but don't know what to do. They can feel helpless. Loved ones can then respond to this sense of helplessness in unfortunate ways.

Here's how it commonly happens. They initially feel bad for you and so they pick up the slack. For example, they do chores at home that you used to do and they willingly do them for a while. The added load is, however, stressful and, over time, they get a little resentful. But then they feel bad about it – how do you square being upset with someone who you love and who is living in pain every day? So, they stuff it and keep going, but the resentment eventually returns and keeps returning. This dilemma leads to stress.

You, the patient, can then feel even more depressed because you see how your situation is affecting them. As a result, you both end up feeling down. You feel guilty and stressed. They feel resentful and stressed, but also guilty for getting resentful towards you! By this point, everyone's feeling stuck and helpless.

It can get worse. Loved ones can respond to their sense of helplessness by taking it in one of two ways. At one extreme, they deny their helplessness and become overly supportive in an attempt to be helpful. At the other extreme, they take out their helplessness on you by becoming overly doubtful of the legitimacy of your pain. You can see these responses on a spectrum like the following:

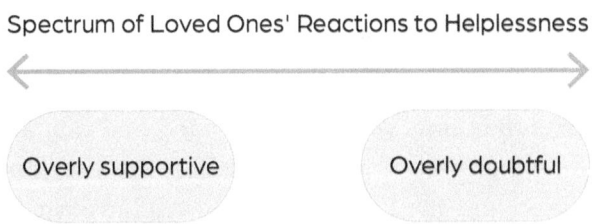

Spectrum of Loved Ones' Reactions to Helplessness

Overly supportive   Overly doubtful

Let's take one at a time.

Sometimes, loved ones, like spouses or significant others, tend to compensate for their sense of helplessness by trying too hard and becoming overly supportive. They're typically caretakers at heart. They tend to feel good about themselves by helping others feel good. As such, they volunteer to do things that the patient can do and discourage the patient from doing things out of concern that pain might increase. They might repetitively admonish the patient, "Oh, honey, don't do that... I'll do that." They might also encourage patients to rest more or take more medications. Their intention is to be helpful.

But is it?

You're trying to keep from letting pain control you. You're trying to do more, rest less, and take less medication. You're working on becoming less dependent, not allowing others to do things for you. If you have a spouse or other loved one, who is overly supportive, it's important to intervene and get on the same page.

There are a number of things you might do. First, have a loving and tactful discussion about your rehabilitation goals. Validate their intentions and express appreciation for them. Let them know that you recognize they're trying to be helpful and that you appreciate it. Then, share your rehabilitation goals and that the only way for you to succeed in achieving your goals is for you to practice reaching them, which means you need to do more while practicing managing your pain at the same time.

Second, encourage them to read this book too. It helps to have a common understanding of the plan. In most instances, loved ones who are responding to your pain in these ways haven't yet made the switch to a rehabilitation model of how to get better. They still see your pain as an acute injury or illness for which rest and taking more medications help. By reading the book, you and your loved one can talk about how there was a time and place for that model of care but you now have a chronic condition and the acute medical model just isn't going to get you better – in fact, it'll make you worse.

Third, remind them of the need to reduce pain talk: you'll update them if any important changes in your health occur, but until then you want to keep off the subject.

Fourth, CPRPs encourage loved ones to come in and work on relationship problems with the patient. If you're not in a formal program, discuss with your chronic pain rehabilitation provider the possibility of brief couples or family counseling. Changing these relationship patterns takes time and practice, but it is possible.

The other extreme of the spectrum is often harder to change. It's what occurs when loved ones respond to their sense of helplessness with increasing frustration and irritability, which become doubt of the legitimacy of your pain. It's the persistent doubt that maybe your pain isn't really as bad as you say it is. This relationship pattern leads to conflict and stress (Herbette & Rime, 2004). You come to feel distant from each other as you both hold resentments toward each other. It's a problem.

If your relationship with your spouse or sibling or parent looks like this description, you likely need professional assistance to straighten it out. Usually, the whole topic has become so sensitive that it's hard for you or your loved one to talk about it without starting another argument.

It's helpful to have a neutral third party to facilitate the discussion and ultimately help you both get back on the same page. Ask your CPRP providers about it and come up with a plan to overcome it.

In the meantime, your work towards reducing pain talk and pain behaviors should help. A commitment to talk about the issues of life, rather than your pain, can minimize the expressions of doubtfulness, and it might also remind both of you that there's more to your relationship than just pain. Also, a reduction of pain behaviors reduces still further any opportunity for your loved one to express doubt of the legitimacy of your pain.

Another intervention is to ask your loved one to read this book. It can provide you both with a common understanding of pain and your plan to overcome it, which can lead to increased trust. It might correct your loved one's misperceptions of you, helping them to understand that you really are trying to get better and how you are in fact doing it. As a result, your loved one might just respond to your pain with a little more empathy.

Overcoming relationship problems leads to improved coping with pain. Everything in life is harder to manage when feeling misunderstood. You feel alone and isolated. As such, you feel more vulnerable to the problems of life. If your loved ones are overly supportive, you can be frustrated with them, but also conflicted – what do you do with your frustration when they're trying to be helpful? How do you tell them that they are doing too much for you? If your loved ones have become angry and overly doubtful of the legitimacy of your pain, you become isolated, hurt, and angry too. All of life's problems, including your pain, are now harder to handle.

Once you and your loved one overcome these problems, however, you are no longer so alone, frustrated, hurt, and angry. Once on the same page, you again have a partner to work on the issues of life together.

Notice, then, what happens. Nothing about the problems themselves change but you both change. You move up the coping spectrum. By overcoming relationship problems, all of life's problems – including chronic pain – become less problematic and easier to handle. It's a way to make tolerable what was once intolerable.

Chapter summary

Coping is a subjective response to a problem. While coping can differ from person to person or from time to time, there are common ways that we all cope with problems. Coping can thus be seen as occurring along a spectrum from better to worse. While there are no instruction manuals, we can learn to cope better with problems. By coping better with a problem, the problem comes to be seen as less problematic. In other words, what was once intolerable becomes tolerable: it's a succinct way to state your goal of learning to cope better with chronic pain.

One broad way to cope better with chronic pain is to work on overcoming the secondary stressors that occur because of chronic pain. In this chapter, we reviewed how to overcome anxiety, depression, and recurrent relationship problems. Progress on any or all of these secondary problems can lead to better coping. As coping with pain improves, you find it easier to deal with pain and it becomes less problematic in your life.

CHAPTER SEVEN

Changing Your Specific Subjective Reactions to Pain

In the last chapter, we described in detail the nature of coping and how it's a subjective response to a problem. We reviewed that getting better at coping with a problem leads to the problem becoming, well, less problematic. In other words, by coping better, problems become tolerable.

We introduced this notion as it applies to pain. We reviewed multiple ways to improve your ability to cope with pain by overcoming problems that occur as a result of pain. These secondary stressors were anxiety, depression, and relationship problems. By overcoming these problems, you come to cope better and as a result, the experience of chronic pain becomes increasingly tolerable. As previously stated, we'll discuss in later chapters some more secondary problems, such as disability, which, when overcome, can also help in just this way. In this chapter, let's turn our attention away from problems that occur as a result of pain and focus on how to get better at coping with pain itself.

Coping better is changing your psychological reactions to pain

If we don't know anything about a problem or if we understand it in some inaccurate ways or if we're afraid of it, the problem is pretty hard to deal with. But if we know what the problem is and have seen it many times and are actually well-practiced at dealing with it, then the problem is no longer so bad – it's pretty easy to deal with.

Take, for example, the experience of having a flat tire on the side of a road. If you don't know a thing about cars and have never changed a tire before, the experience of having a flat tire can be fairly overwhelming. The tire blows out while driving and it's a bit of a shock. You subsequently pull over on the side of the road and face the problem of changing the tire as the cars speed by you. Because the whole experience is daunting, you might just whip out your cell phone and call a tow truck, not even bothering to look for the spare tire, jack, and tire iron.

Now, suppose, you have a flat tire, pull over and face the challenge of changing the tire, but in this scenario someone had previously taught you how to change a tire and you had practiced it many times before. The problem of changing a tire on the side of the road while cars speed by you would be pretty easy. It might, of course, be inconvenient or a nuisance, but you wouldn't feel overwhelmed or need to rely on someone else to help – no need to call a tow truck. You'd just do it yourself and move on.

Same problem, two really different experiences.

Here's where we can understand why you're seeing a psychologist for chronic pain and why, historically, CPRPs are psychology-driven programs.

"Huh?" You might say.

Okay, hang in there with me for a moment.

Among healthcare providers, whose scope of practice best includes the two prongs of self-management – lifestyle change and increased coping? Psychologists are the experts in behavior change – in getting people to make healthy lifestyle changes to improve their well-being. More importantly, psychologists are the experts in getting people to cope better with problems. After all, coping is ultimately a psychological response to a problem. It's more than overcoming the anxiety or depression that occurs as a result of a real-world problem – like what we discussed in the last chapter. Coping is also our psychological response to the real-world problem itself. In our tire-changing example, we reviewed two very different experiences of the same problem. That is to say, we reviewed two very different psychological responses to the problem. The same event occurred, but there were two different attitudes about changing tires, two different ways of making sense of what was going on, two different levels of confidence in changing a tire, two different emotional reactions, and subsequently two different behaviors. Each individual was coping in their own way, but the two different ways of coping and the component parts of coping are ultimately psychological in nature – attitudes, beliefs, ways of making sense of an issue, self-confidence, emotions, and behaviors.

The same is true for pain and the different reactions to pain across different individuals or within the same individual but across different times.

While you may have never thought about it this way, you've always been having psychological reactions to your pain. You've always had attitudes and beliefs about you and your pain; you've always had ways of making sense of your pain; you've always had varying levels of self-confidence in tolerating pain; you've always had emotional reactions to your pain; and you've always had behavioral responses to your pain – behaviors you do in response to your pain or as a way of managing pain. These are all inherently psychological in nature.

Just as we discussed in the last chapter, these psychological reactions to pain – these attitudes, beliefs, ways of making sense of the issue, self-confidence, emotions, and behaviors – can be more or less helpful in dealing with a problem like pain. We could plot them on our coping spectrum illustration:

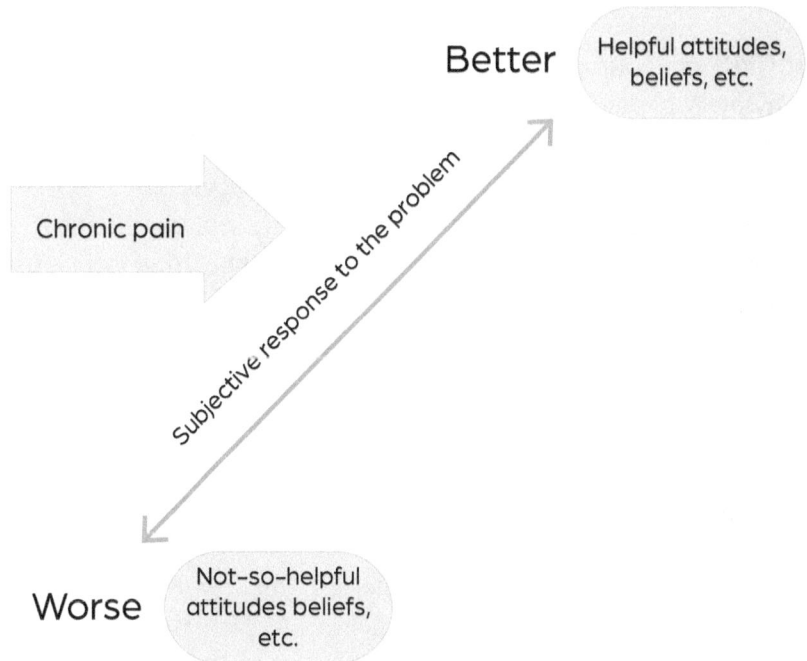

This illustration could be just as much about plotting the different experiences of changing a tire as it is about the different experiences of pain. Just as different psychological reactions to changing the tire made the same problem go from being intolerable to tolerable, so too can changing your psychological reactions to chronic pain make the experience of pain go from intolerable to tolerable.

What this chapter is about – indeed, what this book and what CPRPs are about – is how to improve your psychological responses to pain. We've been calling it lifestyle change and increased coping, but that could also be seen as just shorthand for improved attitudes and beliefs about pain, more accurate understanding of the nature of pain, increased self-confidence in dealing with pain, more empowered emotional reactions to pain, and more healthy behaviors that lead to less pain.

So, let's proceed to work on the heart of the matter – changing your psychological reactions to pain itself (a.k.a., improving how you cope with pain).

Adopting the attitude that you are still healthy when in pain

Most CPRPs encourage patients to adopt an attitude that they remain healthy even if they have chronic pain. We approach patients in this manner: run the following experiment on yourself – take a moment and say to yourself, "I am a healthy person who has chronic pain." Reflect on what comes to mind after you say this statement to yourself.

What's your reaction? Do you consider yourself healthy? Let's assume, for the moment, that you have no chronic illness – such as diabetes or heart disease. The only thing you have is chronic pain – chronic low back or neck pain, fibromyalgia, chronic migraines, complex regional pain syndrome, or some other pain syndrome. Do you see yourself as healthy?

Most patients don't see themselves as healthy. Chronic pain is a health problem, they reason, and as such you go to see a doctor for it. Unhealthy people and sick people see doctors. Sick people take medicines. Pain medications are medicines. As with any illness, there's something medically wrong with you, which produces symptoms. Rather than fever or some other symptom, your symptom is pain. Chronic pain is like having chronic symptoms of any illness. You're unhealthy when having chronic pain. So, you conclude:

Chronic pain = Illness

Sounds reasonable, right?

Let's think about it for a moment. There's a lot at stake here. If you make sense of chronic pain as a health problem, which is on par with an illness or sickness, there are consequences that make it hard to be able to self-manage pain successfully.

First, if you consider yourself ill, what do sick people do? More importantly, what do we think sick people should do? Well, rest and stay home from work. Second, sick people take medicines to get better. Reacting to your condition as if it's an illness leads to resting, staying home from work, and taking medicines. This approach is all well and good if your condition is strep throat. It will likely help you to get better.

But what if your condition is chronic pain? What do you think then? You react to chronic pain by chronically resting, which leads to de-conditioning and increased pain; you chronically stay home from work, which leads to disability; you chronically take medicines in order to get better, which leads to becoming dependent on pain medications. Do these long-term consequences really make you better?

By conventional criteria that healthcare providers use to measure the effectiveness of chronic pain management, this strategy is a failure. These criteria are a) does it reduce pain? b) does it help patients return to work? and c) does it help patients become less reliant on the healthcare system? Responding to chronic pain as if it's an illness doesn't make you better by these standard criteria of effectiveness. Rather, you continue to have pain, which is disabling, and for which you remain reliant on the healthcare system.

Now, of course, some patients will answer affirmatively to the previous question of whether they're better off. They might think back to how they were when they initially came to have pain and how they struggled to remain at work. They might compare that previous time with the present and conclude that their pain and life generally are easier to deal with now that they're on disability and taking pain medications. In these cases, I'd still ask whether 'the better' that we're talking about is really good enough. Is staying home on disability and reliant on pain medications really good enough? I doubt it. Otherwise, you wouldn't be reading this book or be in a CPRP.

I'd support your dissatisfaction with these long-term consequences. Don't be satisfied with them. Continue to learn how to self-manage pain. Get into a CPRP, if you haven't already. There's no form of chronic pain management that has better outcomes in terms of being able to return to work and to do so while managing pain without the use of narcotic pain medications. No surgery, injections, narcotic pain medications, or physical therapy alone – none of these forms of pain management have better outcomes than CPRPs. Therefore, don't be satisfied.

So, maybe it's time to re-think how you think about having chronic pain.

I had a relative who had chronic back pain that began with an injury that he sustained in World War II. He lived every day of his adult life in pain and yet he also worked full-time and he didn't take medications for it. He didn't consider himself ill. He might have referred to it on occasion, but when he did, he thought of it as "my old war injury." For him, it was a static condition that wasn't going anywhere, like an old scar, that occurred in the background of his attention to everyday life. This way of thinking about it matters. It didn't rise to the level of a health problem for which he needed to respond with *illness behaviors* – resting, staying home, and taking medicines. He just never thought of it as an illness.

You might know of people who make sense of their chronic pain in similar ways. They think of it as "my old high school football injury," or "my trick knee," or "my bad back." They might consider chronic pain as just part of life or just part of what it means to get older. They maintain an attitude about their chronic pain in ways like they maintain attitudes about other common problems in life that you can't do much about

– like death, rainy days, traffic jams, and the fact that there are obnoxious people in the world. It just doesn't pay to get too upset about any of these things, let alone allow them to stop you in your tracks. People maintain similar attitudes about chronic pain.

In fact, it's common. The prevalence of chronic pain in the general population is between 15-25% (Gureje, et al., 2001; Toblin, et al, 2011). It's safe to assume that 15-25% of the population isn't engaged in illness behaviors or the long-term consequences of disability and reliance on narcotic pain medications. So, how do people do it? In the introduction to this book, I commented that some people just naturally do it while others have to learn. People like my relative just naturally do it and he did it, in part, by maintaining a healthy attitude about himself even though he had chronic pain. You can do it too.

Chronic pain isn't the only biological problem that we tend to put up with by maintaining a similar attitude. They range from the insignificant to the more significant. On one end of the spectrum, we might list skin wrinkles or gray hair, and moving up the spectrum of significance we might list in-grown toenails, boils, and gastrointestinal systems which are sensitive to spicy foods; and on the other end of the spectrum, we might list sebaceous cysts and eczema. While some people, of course, become distressed enough to do something about these things (e.g., ranging from dying hair to plastic surgery), no one really thinks of having these biological problems as an indicator of being unhealthy or feeling the need to respond with illness behaviors. Some people may initially respond to sebaceous cysts or eczema by seeking healthcare, but they soon learn that these conditions aren't dangerous and that there isn't much that can be done for them. As a result, people don't consider themselves to be unhealthy and so don't engage in illness behaviors. They might think of these things as unfortunate or a nuisance, but not as a sign of being unhealthy. They come to have an attitude of putting up with it.

Many people consider living with chronic pain in the same way. They think of it in the same category as a condition that they live with but doesn't rise to the level of making them unhealthy and so they don't engage in illness behaviors as a result. In other words, they maintain an attitude that they're healthy despite having chronic pain.

This attitude is something that you can learn to have. Changing an attitude isn't easy, but it is possible. Usually, our attitudes change subtly and it tends to happen to us as opposed to setting out to intentionally do it. Over time, we get more and more exposed to people who have the attitude and talk in ways that imply or assert the attitude and after a while, we acquire the attitude ourselves. For instance, think of how our attitudes have changed about smoking. Remember when we started to talk about it as being unhealthy? It was cool to smoke at the time, but now it's not. We used to take for granted that people smoked in public places; now we take it for granted that such places are smoke-free. It would strike us as odd if someone lit up in a waiting room or at your work office – though people used to do it all the time and we never thought anything of it. Did we set out to adopt these new attitudes? No, not really. People just started talking and behaving this way and they continued despite having, at first, the sense of it being odd. Over time, we started talking and behaving this way too, and at some point we came to have a different attitude about smoking, the one that we have now.

You can do the same thing by adopting a healthy attitude about having chronic pain, but you can do it more intentionally. Start practicing thinking of yourself as healthy despite having chronic pain. Actually say the words to yourself as often as you can be reminded to do so. Talk about it with your healthcare providers and with the other patients in your CPRP. Talk about it with your loved ones. Have them read this chapter too. Keep at it despite the fact that it might sound sort of odd to you.

Also, expose yourself to people like my relative. Given how common chronic pain is in the population, it's likely that you have such a person in your life. It might be a friend, relative, neighbor, coworker, or an acquaintance in your religious community. Ask them how they manage their pain. Pay attention to how they go about their daily activities. Keep at it, despite any sensitivity you might have in comparing how they respond to their chronic pain and how you've been responding to your chronic pain.

Remember, there's no shame in acknowledging these differences. Some people just naturally play basketball or play a musical instrument well. Some have to learn. There's no shame in being someone who has to work at learning how to play basketball or play an instrument. It just so happens that you're one of those people who has to work at learning to self-manage pain. There's no shame in that.

In these ways, you adopt the attitude that you're a healthy person with chronic pain. Chronic pain is a condition that you've had checked out and have found that there isn't much the healthcare system can do for you. You're going to have to put up with it. You can put up with it in better or worse ways. Changing your attitude about it is an important step in coming to cope better with it. You're not an unhealthy person when having chronic pain. You're not sick. Chronic pain isn't a condition that rises to the level of illness for which you have to respond with illness behaviors like resting, staying home, and taking medicines. In fact, these behaviors don't make you better. So, you conclude:

Chronic pain ≠ Illness

Sound reasonable?

The importance of how you make sense of your pain

Patients commonly come to CPRPs with beliefs about the nature of their pain, which they've learned from healthcare providers. Typically, they believe that there is a clearly defined structural abnormality that is causing their pain. While there could be structural abnormalities associated with most chronic pain conditions, it would be helpful, in this section, to use an example. Let's use the example of chronic back pain because a) it's the most common type of chronic pain condition which we see in CPRPs and b) among chronic pain conditions, patients are typically most familiar with the structural abnormalities associated with it.

The structural abnormalities that are most commonly cited as responsible for chronic back pain are abnormalities of the spine. In some respects, it stands to reason. People have pain in their back. So, where else are you going to look for the cause of their pain but in the spine? Moreover, there are times when patients report that their pain started with a specific injury to their back – like a sharp pain that started while lifting something heavy. So, again, where else do you look for the cause but in the spine?

There are common abnormalities of the spine that are seen on CT and MRI scans. These abnormalities are a loss of disc height, disc bulges and herniations, annular tears, endplate changes, Schmorl's nodes, nerve impingement (what's called neuroforaminal stenosis), and central canal stenosis, among others. Some healthcare providers, particularly spine surgeons and interventional pain physicians, tend to attribute the cause of back pain to one or more of these findings on CT or MRI scans. In my experience, these types of providers describe to their patients in a fair amount of detail how these abnormalities cause pain. They also describe these details with a high level of confidence that these explanations are accurate. As such, patients tend to be quite confident too that these abnormalities are the cause of chronic back pain.

This confidence seems well-founded. You commonly see these abnormalities on CT and MRI scans. It's right there before your eyes. It doesn't take a rocket scientist to connect the dots and understand these abnormalities as the cause of back pain.

Let's call this way to make sense of back pain 'the structural abnormality hypothesis.' Patients and their healthcare providers, spine surgeons, and interventional pain physicians in particular, often make sense of chronic back pain in this way.

This confidence in the structural abnormality hypothesis, however, can be problematic in a number of ways if you want to self-manage pain successfully.

Pragmatically, this way of making sense of pain leads chronic back pain patients to rely on treatments that have a low probability of success and overlook treatments that have a higher rate of success. Patients tend to seek out procedures, like surgery and interventions, which attempt to repair or otherwise modify the structural abnormalities in the spine. Indeed, these therapies are the most common invasive procedures sought by patients with back pain, and yet, they are the least effective. Reviews of the research by neutral experts conclude that there's only minimal evidence that lumbar surgeries reduce low back pain (Gibson & Waddell, 2007) and there's no evidence that cervical surgeries reduce neck pain (Van Middelkoop, et al., 2012; Nikolaidis, Fouyas, Sandercock, & Statham, 2008). Epidural steroid injections fare no better (Arden et al., 2005; Ng, Chaudhary, & Sell, 2005). Nonetheless, patients seek such care because it seems to make sense that these therapies should work: there's pain in the back; the scans show abnormalities in the spine; so it seems logical to attempt to fix the abnormalities in the spine.

Meanwhile, CPRPs are typically the last thing patients are willing to try and yet they are the most effective (Gatchel & Okifuji, 2006; Henschke, et al., 2005; Karjalainen, et al., 2003; Turk, 2002). This common unwillingness of patients to participate in a CPRP may be due to a simple reason: CPRPs don't seem to make sense to patients. They might understand the exercise component of such programs, but why learn relaxation therapies or how to manage anxiety or stress? What in the world do these things have to do with back pain?

You're starting to get it, though. In Chapter Four, we reviewed the underlying rationale for why CPRPs work so well. Whether it's through lifestyle changes or improved coping, everything you're doing is serving to down-regulate your nervous system and thereby reduce central sensitization. Central sensitization is the underlying physiological basis for your complicated chronic pain syndrome. Let's call this way to make sense of chronic pain 'the central sensitization hypothesis.'

Besides the effectiveness of CPRPs, is there evidence for the central sensitization hypothesis of chronic pain? Central sensitization is actually one of the most growing areas of research within the field. It's increasingly clear that central sensitization is the main factor that makes acute pain become chronic pain, regardless of the structural abnormality that may have started the pain (Giesecke, et al., 2004; Latremoliere & Woolf, 2009; O'Neill, et al., 2007; Phillips & Clauw, 2011; Woolf, 2011).

One of the more interesting findings in all this research supports a long-held notion in CPRPs that was identified in Chapter Two and described in detail in Chapter Four. It's the notion that *what caused your pain is not necessarily the only thing that is now maintaining it.* Baliki, et al., (2006) took MRI scans of patients with chronic low back pain during times when they had two different types of pain in their low backs. The first type of pain was flares of their chronic low back pain. The second type was experimentally induced acute pain in their low back (i.e., the experimenters provoked an altogether different type of pain in their low backs on top of their usual chronic low back pain). They found that the two types of pain produced activity in two different regions of the brain. The experimentally induced acute pain led to activity in a region that has been previously known to be associated with acute pain, even in people without chronic pain. The chronic pain flares produced activity in a part of the brain that's been associated with emotional regulation, among other things. What this means is that there are two pathways, if you will, for acute low back pain and chronic low back pain. Acute pain affects the nervous system in one way and chronic pain affects the nervous system in another way. In other words, when acute pain becomes chronic, a different part of the nervous system takes over, the part that's responsible for emotional regulation.

Doesn't this finding correspond to what we've been saying? You may have had an injury to your low back, say, but over time, in the process of your acute injury becoming chronic pain, the injury no longer is the most important thing to deal with. The whole nervous system itself, including the brain, is now involved in maintaining the chronicity of your pain – even if the original injury to the spine, say, continues. It's not just the injury anymore. The longer pain continues, the more other emotional problems occur, like recurrent sleep disturbance, anxiety, depression, and relationship problems, which then maintain the pain on its chronic course – via up-regulation of the nervous system and its resultant condition of central sensitization.

How you make sense of your chronic pain matters. In large part, how you make sense of it determines what you go on to do about it: at this point, your job isn't to fix a structural abnormality in the spine but to down-regulate your nervous system.

From here we can see why surgical and interventional procedures don't tend to work well, while CPRPs are effective. By the time pain has become chronic, attempts to fix the structural abnormality that started it all tend to fail. These procedures aim to modify the wrong target. It isn't the structural abnormality in the spine that's maintaining pain, but rather the nervous system. The therapy that most effectively targets the nervous system is chronic pain rehabilitation.

It matters, therefore, that you change how you make sense of your pain.

Degenerative disc disease

By this point in your CPRP, most patients will have accepted that they can't fix their pain and so don't see their job as trying to find someone to fix it. It's common, however, that most patients continue to believe the structural abnormality explanation of their chronic back pain. Their providers, especially their surgeons and interventional pain physicians, have consistently explained that they continue to have back pain because of some structural abnormality in the spine. They may have been told that they've lost disc height or that a disc is bulging or herniating or that it's pinching a nerve. They may have been told that they have "arthritis" in their back. In short, patients will have been told that they have *degenerative disc disease.*

We could think of the notion of degenerative disc disease as a specific version of the structural abnormality hypothesis, as it relates to chronic back pain.

A diagnosis of degenerative disc disease is often alarming to patients. It sounds terrible: you have a disease that is degenerating the discs in your spine. It also sounds like it's inevitably going to get worse. Patients frequently express an anxious and helpless fear, "My discs are deteriorating." Often, they will have been told that it runs in families. The implication is that it's genetic, which seems to further imply that there's nothing you can do about it. It's thus natural to become anxious if you have a deteriorating condition for which there is nothing you can do.

It also naturally leads to the belief that you're ill. You have a degenerating disease of the spine for which you think you should stay home, rest and take medicines – things that everyone does when ill.

Another common belief that stems from the notion of degenerative disc disease is that the spine is fragile. The pain that occurs with everyday activities seems to back this up. It hurts to engage in normal activities and even simple movement can hurt. The pain is a constant reminder that something is degenerating the discs in the spine. It's easy to conclude that the normal activities of life are going to make the degenerative disc disease worse as evidenced by the pain you feel and that the best way to guard against the process of degeneration is to stop engaging in the activities of life.

What happens, though, when you stop engaging in life? You rest and remain inactive. You stay home. You take pain medications. In other words, you engage in illness behaviors. As we've seen, when done on a chronic basis, these behaviors lead to becoming de-conditioned, disabled, and dependent on pain medications. Has it really helped you to make sense of your pain in this way?

The answer is, of course, "No, not really," but the question seems unfair. It assumes that you've made a choice to conceptualize your chronic back pain with the notion of degenerative disc disease. More likely, you were never really given a choice. You were never given another option of how to make sense of why you have chronic pain. This book and your CPRP providers are now giving you a different way to understand why you have chronic pain. It's the notion of central sensitization. It also explains how you've come to have all the other secondary problems that occur as a result of chronic pain.

Now, at this point, patients in a CPRP inevitably speak up, being torn between the structural abnormality hypothesis, and its specific version for back pain – degenerative disc disease, on the one hand, and the central sensitization hypothesis, on the other hand. They might ask, "OK, I get it… If I think of myself as having degenerative disc disease it can lead to unhelpful things like being inactive and getting out of shape, but what I can do is to start exercising and get more active – which is what everyone's been telling me to do, anyway. But nothing you've said has shown that the notion of degenerative disc disease is untrue. I mean, it's still true that I have degenerative disc disease – it's there in plain sight on my MRI." Another common sentiment is something like, "Why does it have to be one or the other? I mean, couldn't it be true that what started my pain is the degenerative changes, which remain to this day, but that I have also developed central sensitization now that it's chronic?" Both are good questions.

Both points can at times be true. There are times when an abnormality of the spine, like nerve root impingement, can be painful. As such, there are times that some abnormality of the spine might be involved in the onset of pain, but then the pain becomes more complicated by central sensitization, thus becoming a complicated chronic pain syndrome. This scenario is one of the many ways which exemplifies the central tenet of chronic pain rehabilitation – what initially caused your pain is not now the only thing that is maintaining it.

The truth is, however, that chronic pain can get started and maintained in a chronic cycle in many ways – including chronic back pain. Degenerative changes are just one way out of many. In fact, the science shows that the notion of degenerative disc disease is over-emphasized in our healthcare system. The explanation can't be true as often as we think it is. In other words, the notion of degenerative disc disease as an explanation for chronic back pain is at least as misleading as it is explanatory.

Let's unpack what we just said. In what follows, we'll review the scientific literature on degenerative disc disease and we'll see that a) degenerative disc disease isn't always painful, and in fact is commonly not painful; b) that patients can have chronic back pain without any corresponding degenerative disc disease; and c) that degenerative disc disease isn't inevitably degenerative and can in fact stay the same or get better. Let's review each of these findings one at a time.

Degenerative disc disease is common and commonly not painful. It goes without saying that our understanding of the structural abnormalities of the spine – what we call degenerative disc disease – has been aided by the advent of MRI scans. There are literally countless MRI research studies of the spine and its possible abnormalities. Among these studies, a number of them have set out to determine how commonly degenerative disc disease occurs in people who have never had back pain.

Why is it important to know the rates of degenerative disc disease in people without back pain? It's important because it lets us know how confident to be when we assume that findings on MRI are the cause of back pain. If structural abnormalities, as seen by MRIs, only occur in patients with back pain, then we can be confident that the findings on MRI are in fact the cause of back pain. But, if structural abnormalities occur just as often or even more often in people without back pain, then the presence of such abnormalities in people with back pain isn't so unique. We might not be so confident that the abnormality is the cause of back pain. Thus, it's an important question to research: namely, what's the rate of degenerative disc disease in people without back pain?

Powell, Szypryt, Wilson, Symonds, and Worthington (1986) looked at this question and published it in the Lancet, one of the most respected medical journals in the world. They had 302 women with no history of back pain undergo MRI scans of the lumbar spine (i.e., low back). What they found was that even in people with no history of back pain, degenerative disc disease is common and becomes more common as people get older. In their study, more than a third of women aged 18 to 40 had at least one degenerative disc and the prevalence went up for those older than 40 years of age. This study was essentially repeated with both men and women and published in 1994 in another flagship medical journal, the New England Journal of Medicine (Jensen, et al., 1994). In this study, 64% of people without a history of back pain had degenerative changes at one disc and 38% had degenerative changes at more than one disc. Takatalo, et al., (2009) performed a similar study on a much larger sample of 558 young men and women ages 20-22 with no history of back pain. They found that almost half of the young men and women had at least one degenerative disc. The results of these studies show that degenerative disc disease is exceptionally common and it is commonly not painful.

One might argue that these studies are finding degenerative changes of the spine that have been pre-existing for some time and as such these long-standing degenerative changes may not be painful. However, what might be painful are degenerative changes that occur acutely, such as a disc bulge or herniation, which occurs as a result of an injury. These might be the type of degenerative changes that are painful.

Jarvik, et al., (2005) looked at this possibility. They had 123 people with no recent history of low back pain undergo MRIs. Three years later they repeated the scans. Next, they correlated any new findings on MRI with new onset of low back pain that the patients had reported in the intervening three years. On the initial scan, when there was no recent history of low back pain, significant findings on MRI were common, ranging from disc herniations occurring in 6% of the group to loss of disc height in 56% of the group. After the three-year period, 67% of the group had had an onset of low back pain. According to the structural abnormality hypothesis, the onset of low back pain should correlate with new structural abnormalities seen on MRI. But that's not what was found. New findings on MRI occurred in less than 10% of the group. These new structural abnormalities didn't correlate with new onset of low back pain at all. The only thing that did correlate with onset of pain was something that the researchers didn't set out to find. The incidental finding was that onset of depression correlated significantly with onset of low back pain. Failing to find evidence to support the structural abnormality hypothesis, this incidental finding inadvertently lends support to the central sensitization hypothesis – that an altered nervous system correlates with low back pain.

Chronic back pain without degenerative disc disease. The previous study also sheds light on the second point we were going to make – that people commonly have back pain in the absence of degenerative disc disease. In the study above, 67% of the sample had an onset of low back pain in the intervening three years yet only a minority of them had any findings of new degenerative disc disease. The majority of new cases of back pain, then, were due to something other than structural abnormalities of the spine.

Savage, Whitehouse, and Roberts (1997) also looked at this issue. They had 149 men undergo MRI scans of the lumbar spine. Sixty-six percent of them had back pain. Of those with back pain, they found that roughly half of them had normal MRI scans. Something other than degenerative disc disease must cause their pain.

While it's common for chronic back pain patients to have no evidence of degenerative disc disease on MRI, to be accurate, we'd have to acknowledge that there's a positive association between having degenerative disc disease and having chronic pain. In their literature review, Endean, Palmer, & Coggon (2011) found statistically significant correlations between all structural abnormalities of the spine and back pain. The associations were weak, however, and they recommended against using MRI as the sole way to determine why someone has pain. What this means is that if you show degenerative changes on MRI, it's likely that your pain is partly attributable to those changes, but they play only a minor role in why you have pain. These findings make clear that there are other causes of back pain, factors that aren't captured by MRI scans.

So, let's sum up what we've learned. First, degenerative disc disease is commonly not painful. It's common to find degenerative disc disease in people with no history of back pain. In fact, we might argue that the majority of the time degenerative disc disease isn't painful. In the studies cited above, 50% or more of the subjects had degenerative changes in the spine and yet they had no pain symptoms. Since we know that the number of people without back pain far outnumbers the number of people with back pain, we can safely argue that the number of people with asymptomatic degenerative disc disease outnumbers those that have degenerative disc disease with symptoms.

Second, a large percentage of people with back pain don't have degenerative disc disease. The association between degenerative disc disease and pain is weak and points to the fact that additional variables must be at work when someone has back pain.

More accurate understanding leads to improved coping. So, how does knowing this stuff help you to cope? How you make sense of your pain matters. Knowing that degenerative disc disease is commonly not painful and that you can have back pain without degenerative disc disease fosters a sense of openness to the fact that there must be more to the picture as to why chronic back pain occurs. It sheds light on the other explanation for why we can have back pain. It sheds light on the importance of down-regulating your nervous system and overcoming the secondary problems associated with living with chronic pain.

Also, knowing these facts about degenerative disc disease makes the average patient with degenerative changes of the spine a little more normal. Should we really call it a "disease" when the majority of the time it causes no symptoms? Whether you have back pain or not, most of us, by the time we're age 40, say, will have degenerative changes in the spine. Many in healthcare argue that degenerative changes of the spine are not, per se, a disease at all, but rather a condition of aging. Most of the time it isn't problematic and, even when it is, it only partially explains why someone has back pain.

With this knowledge, it's easier to maintain an attitude that you're healthy. You have chronic pain and your MRI findings may or may not partially explain why you have pain. Many people, whether they have pain or not, have similar findings as you on MRI. It doesn't seem so odd now to say that you're a healthy person with chronic pain.

This understanding of degenerative changes in the spine also helps to take the fear out of it. Dare we say that, by a certain age, having degenerative changes of the spine is normal? As we've seen, 50% of otherwise healthy 20-22 year olds have at least one degenerative disc and the rate goes up from there as we age even in people who have never had back pain. As such, assuming that you have findings of degenerative disc changes on your MRI, you have findings that other people in the general population have. Seen from this perspective, your findings don't have to be alarming or depressing.

Now, when I talk like this in the CPRP groups, patients start to object in various ways. For example, they respond by asserting that their degenerative changes are progressively worsening or that their degenerative changes are likely worse than others.

Degenerative disc disease is not inevitably degenerative. Let's now look at what happens to degenerative disc disease over time. For after all, many patients have degenerative changes in their spine as evidenced by their scans and it'll be helpful to know something about what it means if you do – other than that it's common in the normal population and that at best it only partially explains why you have back pain.

So, what does science tell us about degenerative changes over time? Do such changes inevitably worsen? And what happens to severe degenerative changes?

Symmons, van Hemert, Vandenbroucke, and Valkenburg (1991) attempted to answer the first question. They looked at X-rays of 742 women aged 45 or older and then repeated the X-rays 8 to 11 years later. They separated the women into two groups, those with back pain and those without back pain. As expected, they found degenerative changes in both groups. They also found that degenerative changes progressed most often in those with back pain. Over the study period, they found that almost 60% of women with back pain had a progression of their degenerative changes; whereas, a little more than 30% of women without back pain had such a progression. Notice, however, that progression of degenerative disc disease isn't inevitable. The remaining 40% of those with back pain had degenerative disc disease that did not get worse. The remaining 70% of the women without back pain had degenerative disc disease that did not get worse.

This study relied on X-rays, rather than the more accurate CT or MRI scans. Is there evidence of the same findings with the more accurate scans?

Using MRI scans on a repeated basis, Matsubara, et al., (1995) followed 32 patients with herniated discs in their lumbar spine and found that, over the course of a year, 62% of disc herniations spontaneously reduced in size and the remaining 38% herniations did not become worse. Here we see a significant degenerative disc problem – herniations – not getting worse at all and in fact the majority of the time they get better. These researchers also found data that pertains to the severity of disc herniations. Contrary to the common belief that the worst disc problems tend to get worse, they found that the larger the disc herniation, the more it reduced.

Another spinal abnormality considered to be degenerative disc disease is endplate changes. Hutton, Baker, Powell, and Sharp (2011) reviewed two groups of patients with lumbar-related endplate changes who had had MRIs repeated over time. The first group was 36 patients with a low level of endplate changes and the second group was 22 patients with more advanced changes. Of the first group with less significant endplate changes, half remained the same, a little less than half got worse, and two patients returned back to normal. Of the second group with advanced changes, most remained the same, some got better and none got worse. Here again, we see two important facts about this type of degenerative change. First, in its least advanced stage, sometimes it does get worse, but only less than half the time. Thus, we really can't say it is inevitable that it gets worse. Second, contrary to the notion that more severe back problems always lead to more severe consequences, we see that the advanced stages of endplate changes generally stay the same. Sometimes they get better, but they don't get worse.

Humphreys, et al., (1998) looked at still other structural abnormalities of the spine, which are associated with degenerative disc disease. They found that foraminal stenosis did, in fact, narrow with age but found no progression of disc height, lordosis, or central canal stenosis. So, here again, we find that degenerative changes of the spine are far from inevitably degenerative.

To summarize, we set out to determine the truth of common beliefs that patients have in response to the fact that degenerative disc disease is common in the general population and that it's commonly not painful. These beliefs are that degenerative disc disease is inevitably going to worsen and that severe degenerative changes are always worse in some way. By reviewing what the science tells us about degenerative disc disease, we see that neither of these beliefs are true. While sometimes degenerative changes get worse, most remain the same or get better.

Also, we see evidence that the worse the problem, the more it either stays the same or gets better.

More accurate understanding leads to improved coping. So, how does knowing these facts help you to cope? The notion of degenerative disc disease as it is commonly understood leads to fear-based reactions to pain. The belief that you have chronic pain, which is inevitably going to worsen, is anxiety provoking. But knowing the facts, as you do now, takes the doom and gloom out of a diagnosis of degenerative disc disease.

You now see that having degenerative disc disease at best only partly explains why you have pain. As a consequence, there is cause for optimism. There is a whole host of things that you can do to get better, over and above trying to fix whatever structural abnormality you have in your spine.

You also don't have to live in fear that you're going to inevitably get worse. Degenerative disc disease isn't the only reason you have pain and even if it was it doesn't inevitably get worse. Take that to heart. Start practicing having the confidence that whatever is seen on your MRI scan is what it is and you are now getting better. Chronic pain rehabilitation is the slow but sure way of getting better.

Moreover, an understanding that degenerative changes aren't inevitably going to worsen helps you to have confidence that your spine isn't fragile. Normal activities of life aren't going to make you worse. Of course, you have to be reasonable about what counts as a normal activity in life. We don't want to count water skiing, jackhammering, or dirt bike racing as normal activities of life. However, dressing yourself, cooking, cleaning, and many flexible work activities can be done safely and should be done. As we've seen, far from making you worse, re-engaging in the normal activities of life makes you better.

Remember that the human spine has evolved over millennia and it has served us well. For most of human existence, we didn't have MRIs or any understanding of degenerative disc disease, let alone the one we have been trying to dispel with our review of the scientific literature. As such, for most of human existence, we haven't thought of the spine as fragile. People didn't respond to chronic back pain by stopping life's activities out of concern that they were going to make their underlying back problem worse. They couldn't if they were going to survive.

And yet, no catastrophic health-related consequences occurred. Reports of the plague and other mass illnesses survive history, of course, but there are no reports of masses of people suffering adverse consequences of failing to stop their usual activities of life when having chronic back pain. Now, there are in fact historical reports of chronic back pain (cf., Allen & Waddell, 1989). However, there is no historical evidence that large numbers of people suffered consequences of not having MRI scans and not knowing about degenerative disc disease or not "knowing" they should stop their usual activities of life. No, by all historical reports, people with chronic back pain kept living their life and nothing out of the ordinary happened to them.

As long as you are reasonable about it, you too can keep living life, or get back to living life, and you can be assured that it won't make you worse. In fact, it's one of the ways you're going to get better.

Adopting this attitude takes work. Remember that we defined coping as a subjective response to a problem. The usual subjective response to pain is a reaction of *fear-avoidance*: conceptualizing back pain, say, as the result of an underlying condition of your spine that makes it fragile and which is inevitably going to get worse; given this way of understanding your pain it's natural to avoid things that increase pain because of the thought that those things will make your fragile spine worse. From this way of making sense of the problem, pain is a sign that the activity is making your underlying degenerative disc disease worse. But now you know the truth. You can begin to counter these automatic reactions to pain. In other words, you can begin to change your subjective response to pain and activities and improve how you cope. However, like any other automatic thought, you have to practice changing it. How do you do that?

Practice catching yourself in the thought that the pain you feel when engaged in activities is a sign that your degenerative disc disease is getting worse. Suppose, for example, you say to yourself, "I can't even get dressed anymore, it's gotten so much worse!" It's a common way to understand pain and it naturally leads to distress and poor coping. Now, though, knowing what you know, you observe these habitual fear-based ways of understanding your pain. After you catch yourself, challenge this way of thinking and remind yourself of what you know – that your degenerative disc disease at best only partly explains why you have pain and it isn't inevitably going to worsen. Reassure yourself that your spine isn't fragile. Remind yourself that engaging in the normal activities of life is unlikely to make you worse: what's more likely to make you worse is stopping the activities of life and engaging in illness behaviors. You know that such fear-avoidant reactions lead to inactivity, de-conditioning, disability, and reliance on pain medications.

So, practice having confidence that engaging in the normal activities of life will make you better. Of course, when you get back out into life you can in fact have other injuries. But, science also tells us that even accidents and injuries, like lifting injuries, traffic accidents, and the like, don't typically make degenerative disc disease worse. Carragee, Alamin, Cheng, Franklin, and Hurwitz (2006) gave MRIs to 200 working adults without any history of low back pain and then repeated the scans every six months for five years. They also kept track of different injuries and accidents that occurred in the intervening five years. Examples of injuries and accidents that they tracked were sports and lifting injuries, traffic accidents, slips, and falls. They found that there was no association between these kinds of injuries and the progression of pre-existing degenerative disc disease. Specifically, as long as the injury or accident wasn't so severe that it caused bone fracture or joint dislocation, everyday accidents and injuries didn't cause pre-existing degenerative disc disease to worsen.

When reviewing this study, patients almost always speak up and ask, "How can this be?" They go on to explain that their pain started when they had a slip and fall, or a lifting injury, or a motor vehicle accident, and the MRI that they had following the injury showed degenerative changes. They go on to say that the MRI plainly showed the damage that the injury caused!

It's understandable that they hold this line of reasoning. Many healthcare providers, particularly surgeons and interventional pain physicians, commonly attribute the cause of what they see on an MRI to the accident, which the patient had. They can be quite confident too when discussing these things with patients and so it's understandable when patients believe it too.

It's a sensitive issue, but hang in there and let's review it, because you might just come to agree that the line of reasoning, which healthcare providers commonly use, might not hold up on closer inspection.

When providers see degenerative disc disease on MRI and say that it was caused by an accident or injury that the patient had, it is an assumption. Moreover, it's an assumption that typically can't be verified because they don't have an MRI of the spine prior to the injury. If they did, and if the degenerative change wasn't there before the injury and it's there now, after the injury, then they can be reasonably confident that the injury caused the degenerative changes. But, without knowing whether it was there before the injury, there's no way to be certain that the injury caused the degenerative changes. Remember, the majority of adults have degenerative changes in their spine, whether they have ever had back pain or not. Without knowing what the spine looked like before the injury, we can't ultimately know whether an injury caused the degenerative changes or whether the degenerative changes were there in the first place, as most adults already have some degenerative changes in their spine, particularly in their lumbar spine.

In their study, Carragee, et al., (2006) looked at this line of reasoning. In their sample of 200 working adults, 51 subjects had an onset of low back pain due to injury or accident. Upon re-evaluation, including obtaining an MRI scan, 84% of them had MRIs which remained unchanged, when compared to the MRI scans they had had prior to the injury or accident. Remember, these injuries and accidents were sports and lifting injuries, slips and falls, and motor vehicle accidents. This study echoes the one by Jarvik, et al, (2005), cited above, who performed essentially the same study on 123 patients over a three year period. Their subjects had no recent history of back pain at the beginning of the study, but over the course of the three years, 67% of their sample reported having an onset of back pain. Upon re-evaluation and MRI scanning, only 9% showed any evidence of adverse change in their spine – whether it was the onset of degenerative disc disease or the progression of a pre-existing degenerative disc disease. So, we have good evidence that even normal injuries and accidents don't cause degenerative changes in the spine in the majority of cases.

At this point, I typically ask patients to stop and just think about what we've learned. Most people need a break at this point. What we just learned turns everything that most patients have been told and believe on its head. It takes time to digest. I encourage you to read and re-read these last few sections on degenerative disc disease. Talk about it with friends and relatives and your CPRP providers.

It's important to digest and accept because, when you're trying to cope better with pain itself, how you make sense of the pain matters. The way you conceptualize it is in fact a way of coping – it's a subjective response to a problem. If you make sense of your pain in a catastrophic and inaccurate way – that you have a degenerating condition that is inevitably getting worse and which leaves your spine fragile, it will lead to illness behaviors, which make you worse. So, you have to change how you think about your pain. The pain you feel when engaged in activities isn't a sign that the activities are making your fragile spine worse. Your spine is what it is. Practice reassuring yourself that, as long as you're reasonable about it, your spine will likely stay the way it is.

More ways to get better at coping with pain itself

Now that you know the activities of everyday life won't inevitably make you worse, it's time to do them with confidence. Of course, you'll have pain when you do them. So, let's talk about how you're going to cope with pain when doing activities.

Pain whether or not you do activities

Chronic pain patients tend to avoid doing things because of the pain they'd feel if they did them. It's a way of coping with pain. But how well does this way of coping really work? As we've seen, avoidance leads to illness behaviors which, when done on a chronic basis, make you worse. So, the first thing to do is to begin reminding yourself of this simple fact: doing activities makes you better; chronic avoidance makes you worse.

Use it as an affirmation - a short phrase you say to yourself over and over: "Getting back into life and doing things will make me better." If you engage in prayer, incorporate this focus into your daily prayers. Put sticky notes around your house with this phrase as a reminder. Do anything to keep you focused on it. After all, what you attend to matters. Archers do better when they focus their attention on the target. On what target is your attention focused? If your attention is dominated by fear of pain and avoiding activities, you won't do well and you won't be well. If, however, your attention is dominated by doing activities, you'll do better and be better.

Another thing to consider when finding your determination to get back into life is that you'll have pain whether you stay home or go out to play and work. Either way, you'll have pain.

Staying home, you avoid activities that might lead to more pain, but you still have pain. Commonly, you're also lonely or bored or depressed or lack a meaningful direction in life. Guarding against pain by staying home comes at a price.

Even if it leads to more pain, tell yourself that getting back into life is worth it. Attend the family gathering, go out to eat with friends, start volunteering at church or your favorite local non-profit organization, or begin the process of returning to work. These are some of the things that make life worth living. When you do, you feel good about yourself again. You have camaraderie and community again. Your day has a purpose again. All of these things help you to cope with pain. Patients almost always express fear that their pain will increase if they start doing these things, but the truth is that the rewards of doing these things will actually buffer the pain that you have when you do them. When you feel good about yourself, when you have a sense of belonging, when you're engaged in meaningful and productive activity, when you have a focus for your day, all of these things help you to cope with pain itself.

It's a whole new perspective on your pain. Or rather, you probably already know what I am saying is true. You've just forgotten it. It's a long-lost perspective. How do you cope with pain? You get engaged in life. Surround yourself with people who like you and know you. Get involved in things that are meaningful or where you can contribute to something bigger than you. Be a part of something. Focus your attention on things other than your pain or your problems.

When you engage in life, you have a focus again – and it's not pain. You move on past the pain. It's a way of coping with pain itself.

Pacing yourself

Whether it's doing household chores, recreational activities, volunteering, or going back to work, it's important to accept the necessity of doing things differently. You have to be open to changing how you do things. This openness to change is also a hallmark of coping well with pain.

Frequently, patients report that they tried to do any number of these activities, but found that they couldn't. When we discuss it and explore how they tried and in what ways they were unable to do the activity in question, they almost always report that they tried to engage in the activity as they have in the past. They tried to do it like they did before they had pain and when they tried they had too much pain and so they came to believe that they couldn't engage in the activity any longer. At first blush, it seems reasonable. What else are they going to conclude?

We might, however, ask, "Is how you did the activity before the only way to do it? Is there only one way to do an activity, like chores, social activities, or work? Might there be some wiggle room as to how to do these activities?" Of course, there is.

A colleague of mine used to encourage patients to "work smarter, not harder." What she meant by this statement was that patients need to be open to doing things differently. Just because you once did a certain activity one way doesn't mean it's the only way to do it or even the best way to do it. People who struggle with having to change tend to have difficulty coping with chronic pain. But, it is something that you can learn to do.

One important change is to pace yourself. When doing chores, for instance, it's perfectly okay to break the tasks into manageable chunks. Today, you pick up the family room; tomorrow, you straighten the magazines on the coffee table; the next day you dust. You might also break the chore up in terms of time – you clean the kitchen for fifteen minutes in the morning and fifteen minutes in the afternoon. You can volunteer at church, for example, for an hour, or two hours or four. While working at your desk, you might sit for a while at the computer, and then stand, raising the keyboard onto a makeshift stack of books, so that you can still work at the computer while standing. After a set amount of time, you take a break to diaphragmatically breathe or stretch or walk down the hall and back. There are, of course, countless ways to pace your activities.

Some patients have difficulty learning to pace their activities. They are the perfectionists and workaholics. It's long been observed that perfectionism and workaholism are common among chronic pain patients (cf., Van Houdenhove, 1986). These traits don't lend themselves well to coping with pain. These are the folks who tend to maintain very high standards for themselves: there's one way to do something and it's perfect; if it's not done right, it isn't worth doing; either do it right or don't do it at all. Can you detect a little all-or-nothing thinking here? It's hard to pace yourself when your only options are to do it right or not at all.

In CPRPs, we often bring up the old childhood tale of the tortoise and the hare. Perfectionists and workaholics are like the hare. They sprint or rest in the race called living with chronic pain. They believe they need to either clean the entire house all at once or don't do any cleaning at all. But remember the story: who won the race? It was the slow-moving tortoise. How did the slow-moving tortoise outrun the speedy hare? She did it through pacing. Slow and steady wins the race. In chronic pain rehabilitation, re-engaging in the activities of life is how you cope with pain, and how you do the activities is slow and steady. Slow and steady wins the CPRP race.

When learning to pace, it pays to be open to feedback. Try to take a light-hearted look at yourself; don't take yourself too seriously. Perfectionists will be the first to admit that they aren't perfect. What they need to take to heart, though, is their perceived need for trying to be perfect. It really is an impossible task. Try to catch yourself when you're thinking that you need to do something perfectly. Be open to others who can observe your tendency to think and feel these things. People who know you well can often see you doing it before you see it in yourself.

Once you catch yourself, remind yourself that it's okay to do things well, but not perfectly. Say to yourself, "Good is good enough." When living with chronic pain, good is defined by doing something – not everything and not nothing – just something. Good is good enough. You're trying not to strike out, of course, but you also aren't trying to hit a home run. You are just trying to get it in the ballpark. Good is good enough.

Notice that we're following the same pattern that we have with overcoming other automatic ways of thinking. You first become aware of the type of thinking or behavior and come up with a name for it, like perfectionism or workaholism or all-or-nothing thinking. You use the name to help identify it in the moment. You practice observing it in yourself, saying, "Oh, there I go again." Once you observe it, you can use your observational self to make a different choice. In this situation, you might choose to remind yourself that 'good is good enough' and then choose to do the activity while pacing yourself. Then, you do the whole process over and over again.

Sometimes, patients complain that it takes too much work. It takes so much concentration and energy. It's true. It does take a lot of work. Chronic pain rehabilitation might just be some of the hardest work you ever do. But, it's only hard right now. It gets easier, the more you do it. You also get better at it. It's like practicing anything in life: the more you do it, the better you get at it. And the easier it gets. Just like playing a musical instrument or playing a sport, the more you do it, the easier it gets. Subsequently, it takes less work. It becomes more routine. So, be reassured that at some point it'll become second nature.

Substituting I-can-thinking for I-can't-thinking

As you've previously learned, I-can't-thinking is a common automatic thought among chronic pain patients. It occurs when you tell yourself that you can't do things that, when you think about it, you still can do. It's a hallmark of not coping well.

If you were a little league baseball coach and were trying to teach a kid how to hit, but every time the kid got up to bat, he kept saying to himself, "I can't... I can't... I'll never be able to..." it would soon be obvious that you have to intervene on how he is psyching himself out before continuing to teach him the mechanics of swinging a baseball bat. Right? It's often easier to see these types of automatic thoughts in others than it is in ourselves. With that said, how often do you psych yourself out with I-can't-thinking?

What we're trying to do is to gain some perspective on your I-can't-thinking. So often, it goes by without ever giving it much thought. It just seems obviously true. Our little leaguer just "knows" he can't hit a ball and he doesn't really stop to think about what he's saying to himself until we stop the play and talk to him about it. In doing so, we bring it to his attention.

How often might you say to yourself or others, "I can't get out of the bathtub" or "I can't do the laundry" or "I can't go to the party" or "I can't go back to work" or some other similar statement? If you're like most patients with chronic pain, you might say such things often. They seem obviously true and so you don't give much thought to them.

Despite their apparently obvious truth, might we ask: in what way are they true? Let's be specific. In the previous chapter, we used the example of going to a party and the subsequent I-can't-thinking that went along with it – an individual responding with a statement like, "I can't go to the party." We recognized, however, if we get really specific, a person with chronic pain is able to go to a party. You're able to move your arms and legs and get to most parties, like a family gathering or a neighborhood cookout. Depending on the circumstances, you may need to get a ride back and forth. Even if you needed to be brought in a wheelchair, you could at least get there and hang out with others. Now, you may have pain at the party and you may even have more pain than usual afterward, but physically you're able to get there and socialize.

The point here is two-fold. First, you are physically able to attend a party. When saying something like, "I can't go to the party," the "can't" in the statement doesn't rise to the level of a physical impossibility. It's also not like a deaf person saying, "I can't hear," or a blind person saying, "I can't see." No matter how they tried or how many work-arounds they might arrange, a truly blind person just won't see and a truly deaf person just won't hear. But you're different. If you try to come up with some good work-arounds, you can attend a party. It's possible.

Second, once we recognize that it's possible, it becomes a question of 'how.' How are you going to attend a party? More specifically, it becomes a question of coping. How are you going to cope with the pain while you attend the party? Or how are you going to cope with the pain afterward? The question of how you're going to cope is the central question here – it's really not whether you are or aren't physically able to attend a party, or any other reasonable activity, like bathing, household chores or even work.

Here's the most important point. What we've done by exploring this issue in detail is to come upon a profound insight: "I can't" statements seem to reflect something about your physical abilities, but they really reflect how you're coping. Statements such as "I can't do the laundry," or some other reasonable activity, don't really mean you're unable to do it, but rather mean that you can't cope with the pain if you do the activity. You're able to move your arms and legs and do the activity. What's in question is how you're going to tolerate the pain if you do the activity.

So, we are again back to how you're going to cope with pain itself. And if that's the case, then how helpful is it, really, to say to yourself "I can't" when coping with pain? It's not helpful. In fact, it's a hallmark of poor coping, isn't it? If others were struggling to overcome some issue in life and kept saying to themselves, "I can't," we'd certainly say, "You know, they don't seem to be coping very well" and we'd try to help them. It's essentially the same thing that we'd do with the little leaguer that we discussed above. It's what we're doing with you now. So, this I-can't-thinking needs to change if you want to cope with pain well.

What if you made it a goal that whenever faced with an activity, you try to catch yourself in I-can't-thinking and substitute it with "I can; it's just a matter of how." Now, that's what we'd call good coping.

You would follow the same process that we've discussed before. You practice observing the I-can't-thinking in the moment, and respond with something like, "Oh, there I go again." You then challenge its accuracy. Remind yourself that what it means is not that you're unable to do the activity in question, but that you might not know how to do it while managing your pain at a tolerable level. So, you make it a point to do something different. You intentionally decide to say to yourself, "I can; I just need to figure out how." Maybe, you think of the two prongs of self-management. You engage in lifestyle activities, which will help – maybe some extra stretching, relaxation, or a walk, or you pace yourself. You also focus on the second prong – how you're coping with pain. Maybe you remind yourself of what you know – normal activities won't make the underlying problem worse; you're a healthy person with pain; you're trying to stay grounded in the presence of pain, refraining from catastrophizing about it or otherwise worrying about it. You also tell yourself that you're open to trying and that you can do these things. Practice having self-confidence. Practice believing in yourself again. It's what good coping looks like.

Ignoring the check-engine light

We mentioned the two prongs of self-management just now. The two prongs are a) lifestyle changes which when done over time will reduce pain through down-regulating the nervous system and thereby reducing central sensitization; and b) increasing your ability to cope with the pain that remains. When patients first come to CPRPs, they often see the first prong as the most important but as they continue they inevitably come to see that it's really the second prong that is most important. After all, the degree to which you can reduce pain is limited. You have chronic pain and you can reduce it through lifestyle changes, but you won't get rid of it. So, there is always going to be some pain, which you'll have to learn to cope with. However, getting better at coping with pain has no limit. The sky is the limit when it comes to coping. So, the biggest payoff comes from getting better at coping with pain.

You get better at coping with pain by taking the sense of alarm out of pain. You change your emotional reaction to pain. By doing so, you move from being distressed by your pain to staying grounded in the presence of pain and redirecting your attention elsewhere. Pain becomes no longer alarming or a bad thing that needs to be avoided, and becomes something like white noise that no longer attracts your attention. Life holds your attention and pain remains in the background, like white noise.

Let's diagram it using our coping as a subjective response illustration.

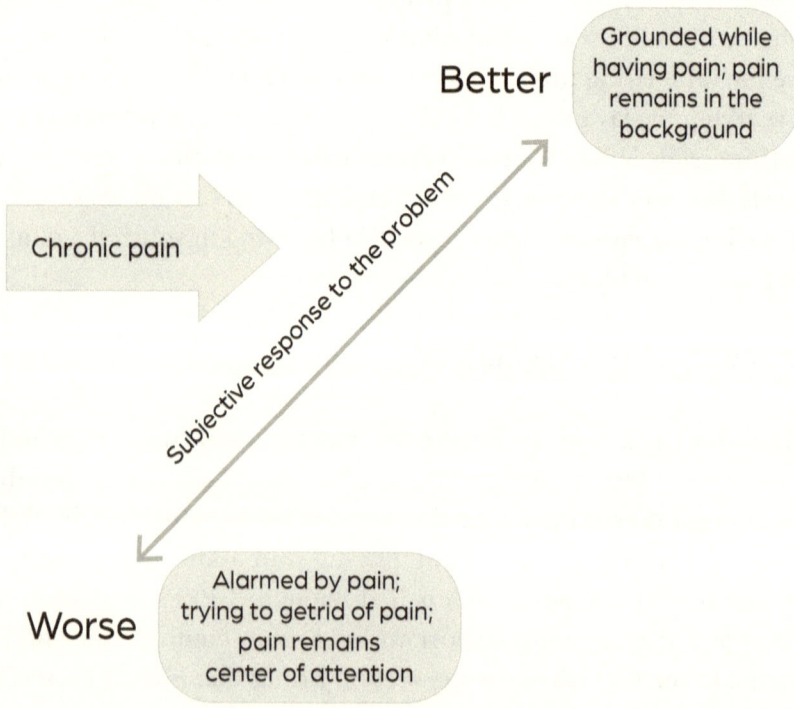

In our diagram, we have one set of subjective responses to pain, which are characterized by alarm and emotional distress, attempts to get rid of pain or otherwise avoid it, and, meanwhile, pain remains the center of attention. It preoccupies your time, attention, energy, and life. These are the characteristics of not coping well. As such, chronic pain remains intolerable. We note its intolerable degree by placing this way of coping below pain on the coping spectrum.

Moving up the spectrum, we have a set of subjective responses to pain, which are characterized by taking the alarm out of pain. You remain emotionally grounded despite having pain, fully accepting that it can't be gotten rid of, fully accepting that it doesn't have to be avoided at all costs, and getting engaged in the activities of life. Pain remains, but it's relegated to the background of life. The activities of life are what hold your attention, not your unfixable pain. It continues, of course, but just as white noise continues in the background. In other words, chronic pain becomes and remains tolerable and so we place this level of coping above pain on the coping spectrum.

In CPRPs, we use a helpful metaphor to achieve this level of coping: pain is like a broken check-engine light on the dashboard of your car.

Remember in Chapter Four we discussed that pain has a function. It's a danger signal that something is wrong. In other words, it's a warning signal. As such, it is naturally alarming and so emotionally distressing. It impels us to action: seek help, guard against re-injury, rest, stay home from work, among other things. The upshot here is that pain is a warning signal, which alarms us and leads us to stop what we're doing.

It's like a check-engine light on the dashboard of a car. Just like pain, the check-engine light signals to us that something is wrong and we become alarmed and we pull over, check under the hood, or seek professional help – we bring the car to the mechanic. This set of responses is all well and good when, like acute pain, it's the first time it happens. You stop driving and get some help and try to fix it.

But what would happen if, like chronic pain, you had checked it out with a number of mechanics who initially tried a number of different fixes but ultimately concluded that there was nothing they could do to fix it? Maybe one or more of the mechanics said to you that there's something wrong with the engine, but nothing life-threatening, and you can in fact keep driving safely. Their advice was to just learn to live with it – just ignore it and keep driving with the check-engine light on.

It would be easier said than done at first. Each time you get in the car and drive off, you have a sense of alarm that you should really stop driving, pull over and get it checked out. But, you remind yourself that it has been checked out many times and there is nothing that can be done and it is safe to keep driving. After a while, you would stop noticing the check-engine light. It would still be on, of course, but you wouldn't pay much attention to it. It would just be in the background, so to speak.

Chronic pain is just like the check-engine light that remains on. It is signaling that something is wrong, but what's wrong isn't fixable. You had it checked out numerous times and have likely attempted to fix it in any number of ways. You've been told to learn to live with it, but it's easier said than done. Over time, though, you come to learn that you don't have to keep stopping what you're doing or go to yet another healthcare provider. Just like with your check-engine light, you start ignoring your pain. You don't have to be alarmed by its warning signal. You aren't making it up, the light is signaling that something is wrong, but it isn't something that you can fix and you have been reassured that it is safe to keep living life. Remind yourself of what we learned about, say, degenerative disc changes. It's safe to keep living life – to keep driving – as long as you're reasonable about what you do. You don't have to be alarmed by pain anymore. It's time to practice staying grounded despite pain.

From victim to empowerment and confidence

People who self-manage pain well have certain characteristics. They respond to pain without alarm and typically think things like, "I have to do my walking today" or "I have to get on top of my stress." Notice how pain doesn't emotionally upset them. They stay grounded. They don't understand the pain as a sign that the underlying condition is worsening; it isn't considered worthy of having it evaluated again; and it isn't seen as a sign of how depressing and hopeless life is. They simply aren't alarmed by it in any way.

They also respond to it with things that they can do. Notice how active of a stance they take. They get out for a walk or they actively manage their stress. They feel in control and empowered to stay on top of it.

People who don't cope with pain well do the opposite. They attribute pain to things they have no control over and so feel helpless and then feel the whole host of feelings that go along with this sense of helplessness.

People who cope well with pain see exercise as a good thing that they want to do. They see pain as the result of not moving. You might know people like this – they say things like, "Oh, I've been sitting too long" or "I didn't get to my walk today." They react to pain by thinking that they've been resting too much. Think about that. They recognize that the body is made to move.

People who cope with pain well engage in activities as a way to manage pain. Activities aren't what they do once their pain is managed; activities are what they do to manage pain itself. Good copers thus respond to pain by getting involved in some activity. They do something to get their attention off the pain. They also feel productive. Subsequently, they are now coping well and their pain becomes tolerable.

Notice how powerful coping can be. People who cope well aren't helpless to pain. Pain doesn't get to them. They aren't alarmed by it. They don't rest or avoid life because of it. Pain isn't a show-stopper. Pain isn't more powerful than them.

In fact, they are empowered. They have the power to affect their pain and their lives. They are in control, not chronic pain.

You too can do it. You're already learning how.

Chapter Summary

In this chapter, we turned our attention to how to cope with pain itself. We encouraged you to adopt the attitude that you're a healthy person with chronic pain. We saw that chronic pain doesn't have to be considered an illness. Indeed, when considered an illness, it leads to behaviors that make you worse when done on a chronic basis. We called these behaviors *illness behaviors* – resting, staying home, and taking narcotic pain medications. Illness behaviors are helpful when having an acute injury or illness, but not when having chronic pain because they lead to de-conditioning, disability, and reliance on medications. So, it's important that you don't consider chronic pain as an illness but rather a condition that you put up with.

Instead of engaging in illness behaviors, we saw that it's best to stay engaged in the activities of life. To be assured that it's okay to engage in activities, however, we had to take a look at one of the most common explanations for why people have chronic pain – degenerative disc disease.

It's commonly understood as a disease, which naturally leads to beliefs that you should engage in illness behaviors. We reviewed what the science tells us about degenerative disc disease. We saw that it's common and commonly not painful. We also saw that the relationship between degenerative changes in the spine and pain in the back is weak and so there must be other reasons why you have chronic back pain. We also saw that degenerative changes don't inevitably get worse. We reviewed research showing that you don't have to conclude that your spine is fragile. Therefore, it's okay to engage in normal, reasonable activities of life.

We saw that people who cope well with pain remain engaged in the activities of life, as long as they are reasonable about it. They pace themselves and are otherwise open to doing things a little differently. We reviewed a helpful metaphor that your pain is like a check-engine light on the dashboard of your car: you have brought your car to numerous mechanics who have assured you that it's safe to drive. Their advice is to ignore the check engine light. You don't have to stop, pull over and bring the car into the mechanic every time the check-engine light comes on. As long as you're reasonable about it, you can keep driving. In fact, it's helpful to keep driving – living life – in order to cope with pain. By getting active, you have a focus for your day. You have interesting activities to do. You feel productive. You feel like you are getting somewhere in life. All these things allow you to cope with pain itself. So, take charge. Empower yourself. These are the active things that people who cope well with pain do. You can do it too with practice, coaching, and the encouragement that you get in your CPRP.

CHAPTER EIGHT

Why You Might Learn to Self-Manage Pain Without the Use of Narcotic Pain Medications

Many patients welcome the notion of learning to self-manage pain without the use of daily narcotic medications. For others, however, this notion is quite threatening. They might dismiss the notion out of hand, as ridiculously impossible, and take it as evidence of my incompetence that I'd even suggest it's possible. The only thing that comes to mind for them is the prospect of intolerable levels of pain and suffering. Still, other times, patients react with feelings of invalidation and anger – as if to raise the notion of managing chronic pain without narcotic pain medications is simply evidence that I don't understand how bad their pain really is. It's not uncommon for patients to angrily react, "If you had my pain, you'd understand!" Still other patients react to discussions of the notion with feelings of shame. They already feel bad about themselves for relying on such medications, but don't know how to manage their pain without them; so when the topic comes up, they feel even worse about themselves, as if they're already supposed to know how to do it, but don't, and so become ashamed of themselves.

Obviously, it's a sensitive issue. But before you react in any of these ways, I'd ask that you hear me out.

Whether you learn to self-manage pain without the use of narcotic pain medications will ultimately be a decision that you make with the healthcare provider who prescribes them. But I'd ask that you read this chapter and consider what you read. Discuss it with your loved ones. If you're okay with it, let them read this chapter too. I'd also encourage you to talk about it with your providers in your CPRP.

Patients and healthcare providers alike tend to make decisions about the long-term use of narcotic pain medications for valid, short-term reasons: to alleviate both the immediate level of pain and the strong emotions that so often accompany it – like those described above.

But what might have made sense in the urgency of the immediate moment may not make sense a year or two later – or five to ten years later. So, as you read this chapter, try to observe and challenge the strong emotional reactions that you might have. Try to have an open discussion with your loved ones and your rehabilitation providers about the pros and cons of remaining on long-term narcotic medications.

Maybe, in the end, you'll decide to remain on long-term narcotic medications, for some situations might warrant them. However, even if you do, you'll have made the decision in a thoughtful way, fully understanding the risks and benefits, and based on your best long-term interests, and not on the urgency of the immediate moment.

Now having said that, in what follows, we make the case that patients with chronic pain can learn to manage pain without the use of narcotic medications and that, not only is it possible, it's in the best interests of most chronic pain syndrome patients. In other words, it's possible to self-manage chronic pain without the use of narcotic medications and, for most patients, you'll be better off if you learn how to do it.

We start by reviewing problems associated with the long-term use of narcotic pain medications. The purpose of reviewing these problems is twofold. First, we attempt to foster some degree of concern in the reader who so far has been convinced beyond doubt that the long-term use of narcotic medications is correct. All too often, as described above, patients are quite sensitive about their use of these medications and won't acknowledge any problems with their use. By having this discussion, the hope is to create some degree of thoughtfulness about the continued use of these medications. Second, for those readers who already have misgivings about the use of these medications, the following discussion is intended to confirm your concerns and bolster your decision to learn to self-manage pain without their regular use.

In the next chapter, we'll review strategies for reducing your use when done with the support of your prescribing provider. Any changes in your use of medications should always be done with the full knowledge and support of the provider who prescribes them.

Before proceeding, let's discuss some terms. So far, we've used the phrase "narcotic pain medications" to refer to a type of medication commonly used for the management of pain. The term "narcotic" refers to a group of drugs that are addictive. A more specific term for narcotic pain medications is *opioid* medications. Up until now, we've used the phrase "narcotic pain medications" because it's likely more familiar to the average reader than "opioid pain medications." However, the latter is more technically accurate and common among healthcare providers. As a result, for the remainder of this book, we use the term "opioid medications" or "opioid pain medications." We also use the phrase "opioid management" to refer to the practice of prescribing opioid medications for chronic pain on a long-term basis.

All opioid medications are a natural or synthetic derivative of the opium poppy, which is a flowering plant. Historically, the first drugs derived from the opium poppy were morphine and heroin. Of course, over the years, heroin was made illegal, but the use of morphine as a prescribed medication continues to this day. All other opioid medications were developed thereafter and now there are synthetic forms of opioids.

Healthcare providers divide opioid medications into two types – short-acting and long-acting. Short-acting opioids are medications that, when ingested, are absorbed at one time. Most short-acting opioids provide pain relief for approximately four hours, with the highest concentration in your system occurring approximately in the second and third hours. Examples of short-acting opioid medications are codeine, hydrocodone, oxycodone, immediate-release morphine sulfate, and hydromorphone. Long-acting opioids were designed to provide pain relief over a greater amount of time. They are opioids that are specially prepared to be extended-release medications. Typically, they reduce pain for about twelve hours, though other preparations are made for pain reduction over a 24-hour period or even longer. Examples of long-acting opioid medications are methadone, morphine sulfate, and oxycodone. Still, other long-acting opioids are prepared in a transdermal patch, or patch placed on the skin, typically to be changed every 72 hours; the most common form of opioid prepared in a transdermal patch is fentanyl.

Problems associated with long-term opioid management

When discussing problems associated with the long-term use of opioid medications, patients most often think of addiction. Addiction is a problem. It occurs much more often than the pharmaceutical industry once would have had us believe. But addiction isn't the only problem and I've found over the years that it isn't very helpful to lead off a discussion about the problematic nature of long-term opioid management with the issue of addiction. Addiction is easily seen by average patients as a problem that lies so outside the norm of their lives that they quickly dismiss it as simply irrelevant to them. As such, patients seem to consider the discussion over, as if, since they obviously aren't an addict, there's nothing more to consider. But again, addiction isn't the only problem associated with the long-term use of opioid medications. We'll talk later about addiction – its definition with regard to opioid pain medications and how common it is, among other issues. However, there are other important problems that we should discuss before returning to the issue of addiction to opioid pain medications.

Tolerance

The first issue is the problem of *tolerance* to opioid medications. Tolerance is when the body becomes adjusted to the use of opioid medications over time and as a result the medication loses its effectiveness. In short, the longer you take an opioid medication for pain the less effective it becomes.

If you've been on an opioid medication for more than a year or so, you'll have likely noticed this phenomenon. At one point, you were prescribed, perhaps, a few hydrocodone per day (or oxycodone, tramadol, or codeine) and it reduced your pain. Over a number of months, you found that it was more helpful to take three per day. As time went on, you found that you needed four per day to maintain the same amount of pain relief. Maybe, at some point, your prescribing provider changed the medication to a different short-acting opioid and that seemed to work well but again only for a period of time. Later, perhaps, you were placed on a long-acting opioid medication, which seemed to work beautifully for a while but the same thing happened with it. At first, it didn't matter because you were on a low dose of these stronger medications and you had room for periodic increases in your dosing. At some point, though, it does come to matter.

Many patients come to a CPRP on moderate to high doses of both short- and long-acting opioid medications and because they've been on opioids for a number of years even their current moderate to high dosing schedule is no longer effective at reducing pain. It's common to hear a history of their medication use that follows the above trajectory – starting on small doses of short-acting opioid medications and over time requiring higher and higher doses to achieve the same level of pain relief. In short, they've become tolerant to opioid medications and it's a problem.

Frequently, patients get referred to a CPRP because their prescribing provider no longer wants to prescribe the medications, as they know the patient is at a dead end. There are conventionally agreed upon upper limits to the amount of opioid medications that can safely be prescribed. So, patients come to a CPRP because they're maxing out on the amount of opioid pain medications that they can take, but the medication no longer works well. These patients are now tolerant to high doses of opioid pain medications and there is no more room to increase their dose.

They come feeling confused and angry that their provider won't prescribe a higher dose. In the past, every time that they needed an increase their provider did so with little fanfare. "Why is my doctor changing the rules now?" they ask. They're angry and desperate, feeling abandoned or betrayed. And while they frequently have a hard time admitting it, they're also fearful of what it means for their future.

Therein lies the problem. Once you're tolerant to opioid medications they no longer work and yet you have the rest of your life to live.

I often encourage patients to consider, before they get to this point of tolerance to the highest doses of opioids, that they need to have these medications available to them in the future so they shouldn't continue down the road of ever-increasing tolerance. What if later in life you are, say, seventy-five years old and you fall and break your hip? What if you need surgery for an unforeseen condition later in life? If you become tolerant to the highest doses of opioids when you're forty-five or fifty-five years old, what will you do later in life? Now, if you have terminal cancer or are already seventy-five or eighty years old, then maybe you aren't going to worry about tolerance. But, if you're any younger or don't have a terminal disease, and are currently taking opioid medications, then you do have to concern yourself with tolerance.

There are really two problems here. First, if you're middle-aged or younger and on long-term opioids (or considering it at the present time), it simply isn't feasible to expect that you can manage your pain with opioids for the rest of your life – assuming a normal life span. Because of tolerance, the medications will simply not work at some point and you'll require doses that are so high that no reputable healthcare provider will prescribe them. So, at some point, you'll need to learn to self-manage pain without its use. It will be considerably easier to taper and learn to self-manage pain if you're on a small daily dose of opioids than if you're on a high or maximum daily dose. Likewise, it will be a whole lot easier if you've been using such medications for a year than if you've been on them for, say, ten years. Second, if you're middle-aged or younger and have become tolerant to high doses of opioid medications (or are on your way to doing so), you place yourself at risk of not having opioid pain medications for future acute medical problems, such as other painful injuries and illnesses or medical procedures. If you're already on the maximum doses of opioids, what will you use for pain relief if you have some unforeseen acute painful medical condition later in life? You won't have strong medications to take that will work for pain.

By becoming tolerant to opioids now, you essentially buy pain relief today at the cost of suffering in the future.

Some patients have difficulty accepting this point and will challenge it. They assert that even if they were (or are already) tolerant and they have an altogether different acute injury or illness, no healthcare provider would allow them to suffer! Would a healthcare provider really refrain from prescribing opioids in such a situation? This common challenge assumes that there will be some type of opioid medication available to be prescribed, but if a patient is tolerant to such medications it really can mean that these medications no longer have the capacity to be effective pain relievers. In other words, it's not a question of whether a healthcare provider will or won't prescribe something. It's a question of whether they'll have anything effective to prescribe.

Now, notice, here, that I'm not talking about addiction. Tolerance and addiction are different things.

They are, however, related. In all likelihood, you'll become tolerant when taking opioid medications on a daily basis for a long enough period of time – even assuming that you never become addicted. If, however, someone does become addicted to opioids, they will also by that time be tolerant, simply because they will have been on such medications for a long period of time. So, if addicted, you'll also be tolerant, but you can be tolerant without being addicted.

At this point, patients often ask, "Well, how long do I have?" There's no definite timeline that occurs. It's different for each individual. Patients become tolerant to high doses of opioids in as little as one to two years or as long as ten to twelve years.

The question implies that the patient is considering kicking the can down the road with the thought that it can be picked up later.

Obviously, patients need to make their own decisions about when to learn to self-manage pain without opioid medications. Here's another instance in which the issue of acceptance comes into play. Patients have to achieve a sufficient degree of acceptance that it isn't feasible to continue on daily opioid medications forever and so come to a point of readiness for change.

It is, however, in your interest to get to this point of readiness sooner rather than later. As stated, the task of tapering and learning to self-manage pain will be easier if you start with a lower rather than a higher dose of daily opioids. Also, it's important for your future that you keep your degree of tolerance to opioid medications as low as possible.

While not fully conclusive, the current research suggests that once tolerant to opioids you'll remain tolerant even after stopping their use for an extended period of time (Chiang, et al., 2010; Lim, et al., 2005; Mao, et al., 2002). This phenomenon has been shown in experimental studies on animals. One study, for instance, provided opioids to rats to the point of tolerance and then tapered them. They subsequently waited a period of time which was the rat equivalent of about ten years for us; they then induced pain and treated it with opioids. The rats required doses that approximated the level at which they took when previously on them (Lim, et al., 2005). In another study, rat pups who were given opioids prenatally showed tolerance to opioids once born (Chiang, et al, 2010). Both these animal studies suggest that other mammals, like humans, will require higher doses of opioids even after an extended period of time of not using them. So, the lesson here is that once tolerant you'll remain tolerant even if you stop the use of such medications for some period of time. As a consequence, it's in the best interest of your future well-being if you get off these medications now so that you can keep your degree of tolerance as low as possible. You want these medications to still work in the future if you have another acute injury, illness, or procedure which is painful.

So far we've been talking about tolerance as a problem associated with long-term opioid management. However, there are other problems too.

Tooth Decay and Loss

One of these problems is the association between long-term opioid use and tooth decay and tooth loss. In chronic pain management, it's not uncommon to see relatively young patients who require extensive dental procedures and even obtaining dentures. As many patients may know, a side effect of opioid medications is dry mouth, or what's called *xerostomia*. Normal amounts of saliva in the mouth protect tooth enamel and with a chronic loss of saliva, there can be a dramatic rise in cavities and tooth loss (Graham & Meechan, 2005; Reece, 2007).

Now, this association between long-term use of opioids and tooth decay is somewhat debatable. Critics maintain that this association comes from experience with methadone maintenance patients as well as people who abuse illegal forms of opioids. They say that the association between the use of such drugs and tooth decay is due to the lifestyles that come along with drug abuse, not the drugs themselves. Such lifestyles, they say, lend themselves to poor dental habits, like failing to regularly brush and floss, and poor nutritional food choices. Now, of course, poor dental and nutritional habits play a role in the cause of cavities and tooth decay generally. There likely is a higher rate of poor dental and nutritional habits among people who abuse illegal forms of opioids or get treatment for such abuse in the form of methadone maintenance. Nonetheless, there's still evidence to suggest that people on long-term opioid medications for a legitimate pain disorder have higher rates of tooth loss (Arneberg, et al., 1992).

Hormonal Changes

Another issue is that chronic use of opioids can lead to changes in the levels of important hormones in the body. In both men and women, long-term use of opioids leads to low levels of testosterone (Vuong, et al., 2010) as well as other hormones, (Katz & Mazer, 2009). This side-effect can cause a number of other problems such as loss of sexual desire, reduced fertility, fatigue, depression, and osteoporosis.

Opioid-Induced Hyperalgesia

Another problem associated with the long-term use of opioid medications for pain is that the medications, when used over time, can actually come to increase pain rather than decrease pain. Most patients won't believe it, but it's true. It's called *opioid-induced hyperalgesia* (Angst & Clark, 2006; Chen, et al., 2009; Hay, et al., 2009; Mitra, 2008; Ram, 2008). "Algesia" means sensitivity to pain and "hyper" is a prefix meaning above, beyond, or excessive. What happens is that when taking opioids over a long period of time patients become more and more sensitive to pain and subsequently experience more pain. So, over time, patients report that their pain is worsening even though tests or other evaluations show no overall change in the underlying condition associated with the pain.

The physiological basis for how opioid-induced hyperalgesia occurs isn't well understood. We might explain it in a general and likely over-simplified way.

Suppose you have chronic back or neck pain. A physiological explanation of the pain is that the nerves in your back or neck send signals to the spinal cord and then up to the brain, where, there, they register as pain in the back or neck. Along this route, there are receptor sites in the nervous system, which receive the signals. You could think of the signals as baseballs that are pitched by the nerves in the back or neck and are caught in a catcher's mitt in the brain. Now, the opioid medications that you take for pain don't chemically act at the source of your pain, for instance, the nerves in your back or neck. As you might think, they aren't stopping the signals from being generated. Keeping with our metaphor, the opioid medications don't stop the pitcher from throwing the baseballs. Rather, they chemically act on the nerves in your brain. In a sense, they dull the catcher's mitt so that the baseballs don't sting so much when they're caught. Now, the catcher's mitt in your brain (i.e., the receptor sites for the signals from your nerves in the back or neck) requires over time more and more of the medication to keep it dulled to the sting of the pitched baseballs (i.e., signals). It's like after some period of time of playing catcher to a pitcher who throws the baseball hard over and over again we come to need more and more padding in our catcher's mitt to keep our hand from stinging.

Now, we don't know exactly why it happens but the medication itself, which in the short term is dulling the receptor site, will, over the long term, make the receptor site more sensitive. So, you seem to need more and more of the medication to keep it dulled, but in reality, the medication itself is making the pain worse by sensitizing the receptor site. It's as if the padding that you've been adding to the catcher's mitt to keep your hand from stinging is actually a rough wool or some other material which over time has come to irritate the skin on your hand, making it more sensitive. At such a point, you have a choice: either keep adding wool to the catcher's mitt, buying short-term relief from the pitched baseballs but making your hand more and more irritated over time; or, you slowly start to reduce the padding, allowing the skin to return to normal, and, paradoxically, have less sting in your hand when catching the baseballs with your catcher's mitt.

Of course, our analogy is over-simplifying a complex process that occurs between the pain-related signals, the nervous system, and the medication. But, the truth is that for many patients, who use opioid medications, the very thing that they are using to reduce pain in the short run is making the problem worse in the long run. This predicament is not unheard of in life. As we've learned, the use of anti-anxiety medications called benzodiazepines can actually make anxiety worse when used on a chronic basis. Also, the chronic use of certain sleeping pills can come to maintain insomnia itself. In everyday life too, we often come across situations where there is 'too much of a good thing.' The long-term use of opioid medications for chronic pain can be one of them.

Mental Cloudiness

A common complaint among patients when taking opioids is the sense that mentally they aren't as sharp as they used to be. Cognitively, they're dulled. They say that their focus and concentration are limited. It's called *mental cloudiness.*

Patients aren't making this stuff up. Research shows that when using opioids on a long-term basis patients tend to have significantly lower scores on measures of concentration, short-term memory, timed performance, and multi-tasking (Kamboj, et al, 2005; Mintzer & Stitzer, 2002; Prosser, et al., 2006).

Psychological Dependence

Yet another issue that deserves discussion is that when patients use opioid pain medications on a long-term basis, they come to have subtle yet strongly held beliefs that lead to a loss of confidence in their own abilities to cope with pain. As a consequence, patients come to rely on the medications long after they stop being helpful. In other words, opioid medications foster psychological dependence.

This issue is difficult to talk about. It's difficult because these beliefs are subtle and don't come to the foreground until actually named, but also because the issue tends to evoke strong emotional reactions. Like any elephant in the room, the loss of confidence that comes with long-term opioid medication use is often overlooked and it's uncomfortable to identify and discuss it outright. But let's try.

Psychological dependence is a set of attitudes that center on the core belief that managing pain well without opioids is impossible. The attitudes that surround this core belief lead to a high degree of sensitivity. In the introduction to this chapter, we described these common, sensitive attitudes. When I question this core belief and recommend to patients that they learn to self-manage pain without the use of opioids, they tend to dismiss the recommendation in various ways. Notice that implied in my recommendation is that managing pain well without opioids is possible and it's this implied notion that patients tend to balk at. It's seen as ridiculous or evidence of professional incompetence. At other times, patients see it as evidence that I simply don't understand what it's like to have chronic pain, accusing me of not having chronic pain. They can also see the recommendation as invalidating the legitimacy of their pain, as if my recommendation is evidence that I don't believe they have as much pain as they do. Notice their core assumption here: managing pain is impossible without opioids and for me to suggest that it is possible really just means that I don't believe they have chronic pain or don't understand the nature of chronic pain. As we've said, it is a sensitive issue.

Where does this sensitivity come from? Does anyone ever get mad at a primary care provider for recommending one treatment over another for a sore throat? Would a cancer patient ever get mad at their oncologist for recommending chemotherapy as opposed to radiation? It must be something about the nature of opioid medications. Antibiotics or chemotherapy simply don't cause patients to become so emotionally invested that they're unwilling or incapable of entertaining any other option.

Opioid medications are different. They seem to foster a loss of this openness. Patients come to adopt the perspective that there simply is no other way to manage pain. As a result, an acquired helplessness sets in. When entertaining the idea of managing pain without opioids, the only thing that comes to mind is intolerable pain and suffering.

Patients are often taken aback when they learn that the majority of people with chronic pain don't manage their pain with opioids.

The prevalence of chronic pain varies among different studies, but a safe estimate is that 15-25% of the general population has chronic pain (Gureje, et al., 2001; Toblin, et al, 2011). It's reasonable to assume that 15-25% of the population isn't taking opioid medications. The research would back us up on this assumption. Breivek, et al. (2006) found in a survey of over 46,000 people in fifteen different European countries that 19% of the general population had chronic pain. In further in-depth interviews of over 4,800 of the respondents, they found that only 5% were taking long-acting opioids and 23% were taking short-acting opioids. So, we can safely say that the majority of people with chronic pain in Europe don't manage their pain with opioid medications. In the United States, the rate of opioid use among patients with chronic pain is similar despite the fact that the use of opioids has become increasingly common over the last few decades. In a study that came out early in the last decade, Fanciulp, et al., found among a sample of more than 25,000 patients seeking care at specialty spine care clinics that only 3.4% of patients were on (or recommended to be on) opioid medications (2002). Later in the last decade, Toblin, et al.,

(2011) found that a quarter of the population had chronic pain, but only 15% of them used prescription opioids to manage their pain.

Now, one might argue that the majority of chronic pain patients should be on opioids and that it's a shame that in this day and age, the majority of chronic pain patients are still being denied the use of such medications. But, that's not what these researchers found when they asked the people in the latter study. They found that 80% of them were satisfied with their pain management. So, it's true that most people with chronic pain manage their pain without opioid medications and are okay in doing so.

The point here is that it's possible. It's possible to manage pain without the use of opioids and in fact, most people with chronic pain commonly do it. They don't have an unquestionable belief that it's impossible. They don't have an acquired sense of helplessness that so often accompanies long-term opioid management. They don't lack confidence in the ability to manage pain on their own. In other words, they aren't psychologically dependent on opioid medications.

Addiction

Before we move on, let's talk about one more issue that concerns the use of opioid medications for pain – addiction. We mentioned it earlier, but let's now go into it in more detail.

In the 1990s and early 2000s, it was a commonly held belief that addiction was largely a non-issue if patients appropriately used their medications to manage pain. Specifically, the belief was that, as long as patients used the medications for pain (as opposed to some other reason, such as to get high), they simply wouldn't get addicted. It was as if to say that as long as one has pain and as long as the intention is to take the medications for pain, then these two factors would disqualify someone from getting addicted. Patients too tended to embrace this sentiment. It was, of course, hugely reassuring. Patients could take these medications for pain and their healthcare providers could prescribe them without any alarming concerns.

But we now know that people can have chronic pain and get addicted to opioid pain medications at the same time. It is not an either-or issue. We also know that addiction can occur in unintended ways. Intentions don't really matter. Indeed, no one ever intends to become addicted to anything, opioid pain medications included. No matter how we slice it, addiction to opioid pain medications can happen. So, we have to be concerned about it.

Let's first define what it means for a chronic pain patient to be addicted to opioid pain medications. A number of years ago, two large professional organizations devoted to research and treatment of chronic pain teamed up to develop and agree upon what it might mean to have both chronic pain and be addicted to opioid pain medications (American Academy of Pain Medicine and the American Pain Society, 1997). They did it because addiction to opioid medications when a patient is prescribed them for legitimate health reasons tends to be a unique situation. In many ways, it's dissimilar to addiction to other drugs or in fact, addiction to illegally obtained opioid medications when not used for pain. To explain, we need to discuss a number of key terms that have been used to define addiction in general. These are the following: *tolerance, physical dependence, withdrawal, loss of control* and *use despite harm.* These are terms that refer to phenomena that are identified and used as criteria for addiction to any type of drug – legal or illegal. That is to say, when a person exhibits these phenomena with regard to some type of drug, we consider them to be addicted.

We have already discussed tolerance, which occurs when the body becomes adjusted to the use of a drug and so you need more of the drug to get the same level of effect. For example, the alcoholic tends to need much more alcohol to become intoxicated than a person who is not an alcoholic (and presumably drinks less often).

Physical dependence and withdrawal are phenomena that tend to go together. They occur when a person consumes a drug for a long period of time. In such cases, you become adjusted to having the drug in your system and it becomes, in effect, the new normal. You therefore become dependent on the drug to maintain this new normal and without the drug, you go into withdrawal. For example, the alcoholic becomes physically dependent on alcohol after a period of persistent use and will need to continue drinking in order to keep from having withdrawal symptoms, such as shakiness. While each addictive drug, whether legal or illegal, prescribed or not prescribed, causes physical dependence, the withdrawal symptoms associated with stopping the use of the drug are different and somewhat unique to each drug.

Now, at this point, the astute reader might think, especially if taking opioid medications for pain, "Gosh, all patients on long-term opioids for pain will become tolerant, physically dependent, and have withdrawal symptoms if they suddenly stop using their medications... Including myself!" True! That's what makes the situation of the chronic pain patient taking opioids for pain unique. The professional organizations noticed this issue too. If chronic pain patients use opioid medications as prescribed for a long enough period of time, they exhibit tolerance, physical dependence, and withdrawal (if they suddenly stop), but we don't necessarily want to say they are addicted in the same sense as we might say it of an alcoholic who has developed the same conditions to alcohol.

So, the professional organizations decided to define a difference between this situation and addiction. They decided to call the above situation *physiological dependence*, a term referring to the constellation of tolerance, physical dependence, and withdrawal. And they decided to define addiction in behavioral terms, specifically *loss of control* over the use of opioid pain medications and continued *use despite harm.*

Loss of control occurs when patients don't use their medications as prescribed or in accordance with the agreements they made with their prescribing provider. For example, we might say that a patient has lost control of his or her use, and so therefore is addicted, when he or she has a pattern of using more of the medication than what is prescribed and so persistently requests refills of the prescription earlier than when it should be due. In these situations, patients often come up with different reasons as to why they're out of their medications early, such as they lost them or the medications were stolen. Other examples of loss of control are getting opioid medications from more than one provider at the same time– multiple emergency room visits and multiple health-care providers, getting medications from friends or family, or buying them outright from people who are not healthcare providers or from the internet. Still, other behaviors that constitute loss of control are altering the long-acting nature of long-acting opioids in order to get the entire dose at once. By doing so, the medication no longer works in a time-released manner and so one gets the entire dose all at once. Another behavior that can occur when losing control is altering a prescription by writing a higher number than what was actually prescribed and then bringing the altered prescription to the pharmacy for filling. When patients find themselves engaged in these behaviors, we diagnose them with opioid addiction.

The other criterion for addiction is continued use of opioids despite the fact that they're causing harm to the patient. When patients engage in the above-noted behaviors, they harm their relationship with their prescribing provider – they break the trust between them as well as the commonly held agreements between the provider and patient about getting medications from only one provider. They can also harm their relationships with friends and family – just as addiction to any drug can do. Patients also place themselves at risk of legal consequences. Some of these activities are illegal, such as obtaining or buying opioid medications from people who aren't healthcare providers or when altering a prescription. Lastly, these behaviors can cause harm because they can lead to accidental overdose. So, when patients lose control over their use of opioid medications, they continue to use the medications despite harm to themselves.

Notice that this definition of addiction is based on behaviors. All patients taking opioid medications on a long-term basis become physiologically dependent and will experience withdrawal if the use is abruptly stopped. But, if patients take their medications as prescribed and take only the medications that are prescribed to them, then we don't consider them addicted. They must display a pattern of behaviors that demonstrate they've lost control over their use and are continuing to use the medications despite harm to themselves.

Now, how often does addiction occur? The research on this issue mostly focuses on the frequency of problematic behaviors like those described above. In an early study, Chabel, et al. (1997) found that about 27% of patients taking opioids exhibited behaviors indicative of losing control. In a more recent article, Martell, et al., (2007) reviewed various research studies that had rates of problematic behaviors ranging from 5-24%.

So, addiction is a problem. As discussed earlier, it was once thought that addiction to opioid medications was rare, but this belief has turned out to be untrue. Patients taking opioid medications need to be concerned about addiction and take the issue seriously. Given all the problems associated with the use of opioid medications, are they worth the risk of addiction too?

Chapter Summary

There is a time and place for everything. The use of opioid medications on a short-term basis can be appropriate, particularly when you have certain acute injuries or illnesses or medical procedures that are painful. When used on a chronic basis, however, they increasingly develop problems that come to outweigh their initial short-term benefit. Because of tolerance, the use of opioid medications for pain isn't sustainable indefinitely – which is a problem if you have a number of years yet to live. They can cause tooth decay and loss. They cause hormonal problems, such as low levels of testosterone. They cause mental cloudiness. They can even make your pain worse over time. They foster psychological dependence. Lastly, a substantial percentage of patients on opioids come to exhibit a pattern of behaviors that are indicative of addiction.

You don't have to agree with every point in this chapter. The goal here is to simply foster a degree of thoughtfulness about your use of opioids and to consider that maybe it's in your long-term interest to learn how to self-manage pain without their use.

The good news here is that it's possible! Most people with chronic pain do it, and you can too. You just have to learn how.

CHAPTER NINE

How to Cope When Tapering Opioid Pain Medications

Learning to self-manage pain without the use of opioid medications can be one of the most empowering things that you do in your life. It's a process of making possible something that was once thought to be impossible and in this process, you find your self-confidence again. Let's talk about how to do it.

Talk with your prescribing provider (and other healthcare providers) first

It's important to note that, before you decide to learn how to self-manage pain without the use of opioids, you need to discuss it with the healthcare provider who is prescribing the medications and your CPRP providers. They're an important part of your team and they need to agree it's in your best interest. There may be health factors that need to be taken into account when making your decision or carrying it out. They also need to support you through the process and to do so they need to agree it's in your best interest. The point here is that you need to make it a mutual decision between you, the provider who's prescribing opioids, and the CPRP staff.

Don't just stop abruptly

Patients often report, when discussing the idea of managing pain without opioids, "I've tried that and it didn't work." When asked how they tried, they commonly say that they abruptly stopped their use and their pain became intolerable. For them, it came down to a simple equation:

no opioids = intolerable pain. It's a no brainer, it seems. But what part of the equation is missing?

There are two important variables missing: 1) they stopped the medications abruptly and so went into acute opioid withdrawal and 2) they didn't substitute anything for the opioids.

If you've been taking opioids on a daily basis for a period of time and you abruptly stop their use, you'll go into opioid withdrawal. Opioid withdrawal consists of a number of symptoms, including anxiety, nausea, diarrhea, runny nose, fever, insomnia, and aches and pain (American Psychiatric Association, 1994). Notice the latter. Opioid withdrawal causes pain – even in those who don't have pain. Moreover, opioid withdrawal is a huge stress on the nervous system – causing anxiety, insomnia, and diarrhea, all of which are indicators of a stressed-out nervous system. This stress is also going to increase the pain that you already have.

When patients have intolerable levels of pain after abruptly stopping opioid medications, they inevitably attribute the level of pain to the sole fact that they are no longer on opioids. In other words, they almost always believe that their pain level at the time is their true level of pain when not taking opioids. They conclude that they absolutely need their medications or otherwise their pain level is intolerable. As a result, they respond to the notion of learning to self-manage pain without opioids with statements like the above, "I've tried that before and it didn't work."

What they don't realize is that, when opioids are stopped abruptly, their pain is amplified beyond what it would be if they simply weren't on the medications. That is to say, even if the medications were effective and so their increased pain was in part attributable to the absence of the medication, it would still be true that their increased pain was also attributable to the fact that they are in withdrawal, which itself causes pain (as it does with everyone – even those without pain), and it is attributable to the stress on the nervous system that the withdrawal causes, which also causes increased pain. So, when in acute opioid withdrawal, patients can have up to three factors causing their increased pain, but patients almost always only consider one of these factors.

Now, having said that, the increased pain can usually be prevented by preventing withdrawal and acquiring other ways to reduce pain and increase coping. So, in CPRPs, we set out with a plan: Slowly reduce opioid medications, which prevents opioid withdrawal, while coaching patients on how to self-manage pain so that they have abilities to reduce pain and increase coping, which substitutes for the use of the medications.

Another possibility to keep in mind is that a large percentage of patients don't have increased pain at all when tapering opioids because of their tolerance to the medication. They don't notice any difference in pain when taking less medication.

Moreover, some patients have less pain. They've been on the medications for so long that their use has been causing opioid-induced hyperalgesia. Prior to coming to a CPRP, they mistakenly attributed their increased pain to a worsening of their overall condition and so took more medications, only to have more pain over time. As they taper their medications in the CPRP they come to find – surprisingly – that they have less pain.

Acceptance and readiness for change, revisited

So where do we start? Like with other things in this book, we start with acceptance and readiness for change. Patients are most successful when they own the need to taper opioids. They come to accept that they can't continue to take opioid medications for the rest of their life and so are ready to taper the medications. Hopefully, the last chapter helped you to accept the necessity of learning to self-manage pain and that you are now ready to do so.

Commit to a taper on a time-scheduled basis

The next thing to do is to commit to a schedule of reductions in your opioid medication use. There are two points here to discuss. Your commitment should be to a series of reductions in opioid use that occurs on a time-scheduled basis and you need to be relatively comfortable with the frequency with which the reductions occur. Let's take these issues one at a time.

What does it mean to reduce opioids on a time-scheduled basis? A time-scheduled reduction is one in which the reductions occur based on an interval of time. An example might be an individual who takes five milligrams of oxycodone four times daily and he commits to reducing one of these tablets each week. So, the first reduction would be to take three tablets per day for a week. The next week he takes two tablets per day and so on until he is no longer taking oxycodone. Let's take another example, one where an individual is at the higher end of the spectrum of opioid use. I once saw a woman over a period of a few years. When I first started seeing her for care she was on a total daily dose of 140 milligrams of methadone, which is a considerably higher dose than what is conventionally considered the maximum dose of methadone. She initially committed to a reduction of five milligrams each month. After a few months, she acknowledged that these reductions weren't making any difference in her pain levels –because of her exceptionally high tolerance – and she re-committed to reducing ten milligrams each month. When she got to the month where she was taking five milligrams twice daily, she went a few months on two and a half milligrams twice daily, and then two months taking two and a half milligrams each day. She subsequently stopped and did well. Obviously, in this latter case, it took her a considerably longer time to taper – partly because she was on a higher daily dose to begin with, but also because the time interval for each reduction was longer. In the first case, the patient made a reduction each week and in the second case, the patient made a reduction each month or even every other month. The basis of these reductions was intervals of time, and these intervals might have been any interval, whether it is every three days, every week, every other week, monthly, or every other month – whatever the patient and the healthcare provider decide. These intervals of time are examples of a time-scheduled basis for tapering opioids.

In a time-scheduled taper, the total amount of tablets that the patient gets prescribed is reduced to reflect the reduced frequency of use. In the example of the individual above who was taking four 5mg tablets of oxycodone per day and reduced to three tablets per day, the total amount of tablets he was prescribed was also reduced. So, for the week that he reduced to three tablets per day, he was prescribed 21 tablets for the week. For the week that he reduced to two tablets per day, he obtained 14 tablets for the week. For the week that he reduced to one tablet per day he obtained 7 tablets for the week. Similar reductions in the amount of tablets prescribed, corresponding to the particular time interval chosen, occur in all time-scheduled tapers.

A time-scheduled basis of tapering is important because it puts patients in the position of having to rely on other methods to manage pain, which they're learning in their CPRP. It's a commitment to not just rely on the pills to manage pain for you. You now have actually fewer medications and you simply must practice the two prongs of your self-management – continued lifestyle changes and increased coping.

The second aspect of committing to a time-scheduled basis of reducing opioids is that you have to be comfortable with the frequency of reduction. Now, of course, "comfortable" is a relative term. Few people are completely gung-ho about it. There is usually some degree of nervousness or fear about reducing, which is normal. It's all part of the process of regaining your self-confidence, by working through the fear and learning that you can in fact self-manage pain on less and less medications.

By the time you start tapering opioids, you should be engaged in regular mild aerobic exercise, daily relaxation exercises, daily hot baths, and reduced caffeine use. You may also be working on reducing insomnia. You have also stopped talking about pain with friends and relatives, and are catching yourself when you engage in pain behaviors. You are practicing maintaining an observational self, catching yourself when you respond to pain in various ways that are unhealthy or unhelpful. By these methods, you are trying to remain grounded when having pain. All these factors substitute for the use of opioid medications and so you aren't helpless in response to the pain.

Don't pursue a contingent-based taper

A common mistake among healthcare providers when tapering patients from opioids is that they take on the task of tapering with what amounts to a plan, which we might call, "a contingent-based" reduction. Basically, what happens is that the prescribing healthcare provider directs the patient to reduce some set amount "if you can," as if there might be times when the patient has less pain and so experiences less need for medication and therefore "can" reduce the use of the medication. To be specific, in a contingent-based taper, the criterion for taking less medication is if or when you have less pain.

This form of tapering makes sense if you have an acute injury or surgical procedure. If, say, you broke your arm or just went through some type of surgery, you might be given a set amount of opioids and told to reduce their use if or when you can. As you heal, you have less pain and you reduce your use as you have less and less pain.

However, chronic pain doesn't fit this trajectory of having less pain over time. If the level of pain is the guide to when to reduce, a contingent-based taper is a setup for failure. To be sure, chronic pain can wax and wane. So, there will be times when patients reduce their use of opioids when having a good pain day, but it's only a matter of time before their pain returns to higher levels and so – letting pain be their guide as to when to reduce opioids – it's inevitable that they return to higher doses of opioids. It just doesn't work for patients with chronic pain.

Tapering opioids is an exposure-based therapy that leads to increased coping with pain

Let's suppose you were afraid of flying. How might you get over this fear? Well, you might first start with seeing a psychologist who shows you various relaxation exercises and introduces you to such notions as catastrophization and all-or-nothing thinking. In the course of the therapy, you practice the relaxation exercises. You also discuss how your fear consists of catastrophized thoughts about the plane crashing and how, in response to these thoughts, you have come up with an all-or-nothing solution – never get on a plane. With time, you start challenging the likelihood of such a catastrophized scenario and discuss alternatives to the either-fly-or-you-don't solution to the fear. In a way, you are following the two prongs of rehabilitation: you're practicing the lifestyle change of relaxation exercises and changing the way you react to, or cope with, the problem of flying. However, learning how to get your nervous system to relax and challenging how you think about flying isn't going to be enough. Ultimately, you have to start practicing these skills in a real-life situation. In other words, you have to get on the plane. The phrase that we use for doing it in a real-life situation is *in vivo*.

Patients with a fear of flying must ultimately practice their skills in vivo – on the plane. To make it easier and more successful, patients do it on a gradual basis. First, they talk about what it would be like to get on a plane and practice their skills of relaxation and altering how they think about flying, but do so in the doctor's office. Second, they later get on the plane and practice these skills, but then get off. Third, they get on the plane, sit down and buckle up, all the while practicing their skills. Fourth, they not only sit down and buckle up, but they actually take off! Fifth, they get on a plane and fly off again. Notice that as they proceed through this process they are gradually exposing themselves to what they fear. We call it *exposure-based therapy*. As you gradually expose yourself to what you fear, you learn both how to overcome the fear and gain the self-confidence that you really can do it.

There's an old saying that if you are thrown from a horse you get right back on. The longer you wait, the scarier it becomes to ride again. This saying captures the essence of an exposure-based therapy. To overcome your fear, you must face what you fear and learn that you can in fact do what you fear doing.

Learning to self-manage pain without the use of opioid medications is also an exposure-based therapy. As patients taper the use of medications, they gradually expose themselves to pain and put themselves in the situation of having to rely on other ways to manage and cope with it. Their CPRP providers coach them through this process. Moreover, as patients do it, they learn that they can in fact do it! They learn, not only how to do it, but learn that they can do it. It's a confidence-building experience.

Learning to self-manage pain is one of the most empowering things that you'll ever do.

Now, at this point, some patients say, "But, I'm not afraid of my pain. I just don't want to have it." This is the acceptance issue again. Of course, you don't want to have pain. But, you have it. There's nothing that can be done about that fact. Even when taking opioids, you still have pain. So, how helpful is it to maintain the attitude that you don't want pain? It's time to stop trying to get rid of it. It's a set-up for persistent failure. What you need to focus on is, not how to get rid of it, but how to cope with it and ultimately cope better with it – because you have it and you can't get rid of it.

As we've seen, many people have chronic pain and they live well. They do it by accepting that they have it and learning to self-manage it. You can too.

You do it by slowly tapering opioid medications, coming face-to-face with what you have been trying to get rid of or otherwise avoid. By doing so, you learn how to cope with it and gain the confidence that you can live with pain and live well.

Remember that the chronic use of opioid medications has drained you of self-confidence and has made you feel vulnerable to pain in ways that other people simply don't feel. Who are these people? They are people with chronic pain who don't manage it with opioid medications. They don't feel as if they have to rely on opioid medications because they don't feel vulnerable to pain. In fact, they just know that they can cope with pain and do it well. You can too.

The only way to do it is to expose yourself to life on fewer and fewer opioids and put into practice what you've been learning. With supportive coaching from your CPRP providers, you learn how to cope with chronic pain and learn that you really can do it.

Tapering opioids is thus an exposure-based therapy. It's a therapy in and of itself. Exposing yourself to pain and learning to self-manage it through participating in a CPRP changes your habitual subjective response to pain – whether it's one of fear or alarm or an attitude of not wanting pain. That is to say, by pursuing chronic pain rehabilitation, including learning to self-manage pain without the use of opioids, patients acquire better and more effective ways to cope with pain. They are no longer afraid or alarmed by pain. They are no longer in a no-win battle to get rid of it. Their subjective response is, 'Well… I never would have chosen it, but now that I got it, I've learned what I need to know in order to deal with it, and it really doesn't get me down anymore. I've moved on and I'm living life." What an altogether different response to the pain! This response is the payoff that you get for your hard work.

This level of improved coping only comes by tapering opioids. I don't believe I have ever seen a patient who takes opioids on a daily basis who didn't lose their self-confidence that they can cope with pain and do it well. I have never seen a patient on long-term opioids who had a take-it-or-leave-it attitude about their medications. As long as you take them on a daily basis, there will always be a tendency to attribute your ability to manage pain to the medication. The medications inevitably come to have the power. They inevitably come to be the source of your ability to manage pain, not you, and you inevitably come to feel vulnerable to pain and reliant on the medication to do it for you. It is only through slowly tapering the medication, coupled with supportive coaching from your CPRP providers, that you learn that you can be the source of this power, that you can in fact cope with pain, and that you can live well despite chronic pain. This change in perspective on chronic pain is simply one of the most important things you can do.

While you can learn a lot before actually starting the tapering process, the most important aspects of learning to self-manage pain can only be done by actually doing it in vivo – which is to say, living life with less and less medication. This point is important because patients commonly want to be able to learn how to self-manage pain, regain their confidence, and *then* taper opioids. However, it doesn't work that way.

If I were a tennis expert, I could teach you a lot about tennis. I could review the rules with you and we could talk about how to hit the ball and where to stand and how to plant your feet. We could also talk about strategies for different types of play. But, if all we did was talk about it and go over charts and illustrations, you wouldn't be able to say that you know how to play or have the self-confidence that you know how to play well. Eventually, you have to pick up a racket and get on the court. Of course, at first, you won't be very good at it. With practice, however, you get better. Over time, you learn how to play and gain the confidence that you can play well. You just can't achieve these goals unless you get on the court and practice.

The same is true for learning to cope with chronic pain. You'll never learn how to self-manage pain without opioids unless tapering opioids is part of the learning process. Of course, it's normal to be apprehensive. However, practice believing in yourself. Other people with chronic pain do it and you can too. Learning to self-manage pain without opioids by slowly tapering your medications and practicing your self-management is an opportunity to take back your life and make it yours again.

Practice changing your subjective responses to pain

As you taper, practice increasing your abilities to cope with pain. Let's review how to do it. First, foster your observational self and observe yourself in the automatic thoughts and reactions to pain that are unique to you. Pain is a naturally distressing experience to have and so it lends itself to fear-based reactions, such as a sense of alarm, catastrophizing, as well as attempts to avoid pain through the illness behaviors of taking medications, staying home, and resting. However, you can re-train these automatic reactions and overcome the fear. You start by fostering an observational self and catching yourself in these reactions and observing them.

Second, once you observe these automatic thoughts and reactions, try to challenge them. In the moment, ask yourself, "How necessary is it that I react this way? Maybe, I can try to change how I am reacting." You might catch yourself reacting to your pain as something that is really bad and unfortunate for you to have, and in ways that lead others to express comfort or sympathy; and so you say to yourself, "There I go again. I don't have to see myself as suffering from this pain. I am not a victim here!"

Or, you might catch yourself catastrophizing, immediately reacting with fear that maybe your doctors didn't diagnose your condition correctly; and so you say to yourself, "I know what this pain is. I have had every test there is and I know what this pain is."

Or, you begin to think about all the things that you need to do, and your next thought is that you can't do anything because of the pain; you catch yourself in I-can't-thinking and say to yourself, "I know that if I pace myself I'll be able to get what I want done. It's just not true that I can't do anything."

Of course, when starting to challenge your automatic thoughts, you won't really believe what you're telling yourself to counteract your automatic thoughts. They're going to just sound like empty words. Your automatic thoughts are so familiar that they seem obviously true. It's hard to break them of this spell.

They are, however, only apparently true. They aren't really true. They are just a habitual way of thinking about your pain. Like with breaking any habit, though, you have to start somewhere. So, catch yourself having automatic thoughts and reactions to pain and challenge them. Have a conversation in your head, putting these automatic thoughts and reactions to the test. Even if you don't fully buy into your challenge, keep saying them to yourself, over and over again. After a while, they won't sound so flat. In fact, over time, they will become the new habitual way of reacting to pain.

When it comes to tapering opioids, one of the most common automatic reactions is I-can't-thinking. As we've seen, the chronic use of opioids inevitably leads to attributing your ability to manage pain to the medications themselves. Over time, you become more and more vulnerable to pain, coming to believe that you must depend on the medications to get by. You lose your self-confidence that you can cope with pain. As such, the persistent theme of your automatic reactions to pain is "I can't cope."

Here again, we can see how therapeutic tapering can really be. With the guidance of your CPRP providers, you make a small reduction in the use of opioids and practice your lifestyle changes and ways of coping. You get some time and practice under your belt. You observe your automatic I-can't-thinking and challenge it. Maybe, you say to yourself, "Other people deal with pain without opioids; I'm no different than they are; I can do it." Surround yourself with people who support you and believe in you. With practice, you come to see that you can do it and you create a little success. Success then breeds success and you see how you might make another reduction in a few days. Each success is also proof that your I-can't-thinking isn't true.

Another focus is to practice having an attitude that you are healthy. Remember, it matters how you make sense of your pain. Tell yourself that you're a healthy person with chronic pain. As such, you don't have to do the things that ill people do – resting, staying home, and taking medications.

Also, catch yourself referring to your opioid medications as "medicine." Pain is not an illness and pain medications are not medicines. Medicines are things that sick people take and they make sick people better. You aren't ill and opioid medications haven't made you better. Opioid medications have made you dependent, vulnerable, and fearful of pain. How you think about pain medications matters when it comes to coping.

Remind yourself of the check-engine light metaphor. You have what amounts to a check-engine light that is stuck on. You have had it checked out numerous times and have had a number of mechanics attempt to fix it and they were unable to fix it. The mechanics have told you that the car is basically safe to drive, as long as you follow the reasonable rules of the road. As such, they have encouraged you to learn to live with it – to keep driving with the check-engine light on.

Similarly, pain isn't something that you have to avoid by taking medications. Every day, people cope with pain by staying engaged in life – staying on the road, so to speak – in a reasonable fashion. Staying engaged in life is one of their chief ways of coping with pain and as such they have ways of coping with pain that substitute for the use of taking opioid medications. By getting back on the road, you achieve the benefits of getting somewhere – you're no longer stuck, going nowhere. By ignoring pain and getting involved in the reasonable activities of life, you are able to cope with pain without the use of opioids.

Notice the active ways of coping that the metaphor contains. Active coping is coping in which you take charge and get involved. Active ways of coping are engaging in lifestyle changes, like regular mild aerobic exercise, relaxation exercises, stress management, pacing yourself, and staying involved and engaged in the activities of life – personal care, household chores, social and recreational activities, religious activities, and most forms of work. These are the things that *active copers* do to self-manage their pain. Passive ways of coping are thinking of yourself as ill, resting, staying home from work, and taking opioid medications. These are the things that *passive copers* do. When tapering opioids, it's important to practice all the active ways of coping.

Common Concerns that Patients Have

Patients, however, want to know what happens if their pain increases once they start tapering opioids. It's a fair question. Most patients, prior to participating in a CPRP, have spent most of their time, energy, and attention trying to get rid of their pain or at least trying to avoid it. Reducing opioids runs counter to either of these approaches.

Now, they might entertain the notion that with tapering some people have little change in their pain level because of tolerance and some people may have less pain because of opioid-induced hyperalgesia, but it simply can't be true of all patients. They think that at least some patients, if not the majority, will have intolerable levels of pain when reducing the use of opioids!

In actual clinical practice, this scenario is rare, at least if we're talking about a situation in which someone's pain becomes intolerable and remains intolerable thereafter. There are times, of course, when patients experience intolerable levels of pain in the course of a CPRP. As staff, we respond to it, making adjustments to their medications, but also by coaching patients on what to do about it and how to respond to it with increased coping skills. As a result, patients come to get a handle on the increased pain and reduce it back down to more tolerable levels. As such, it just doesn't happen that pain will remain intolerable indefinitely once opioids are tapered.

Rather, with teamwork and support, patients come to create a successful experience even with the increased pain that can come with tapering opioids. They learn that they can keep their pain at a tolerable level. They see how self-management can work and it becomes a highly empowering experience for them.

We also remind them, in the course of their participation, that they had times when they experienced intolerable levels of pain, even when they were on opioid medications. One perspective to take is that in this way it is no different. You had pain flares while on opioids and you will have pain flares now that you are working towards getting off opioids. In another way, though, it is different. You are now learning how to cope with pain flares and bring them back down without reaching for more pills.

When patients work at getting good at the lifestyle changes and ways of coping that they learn in a CPRP, they typically reduce their pain or otherwise maintain their pain at the level it was when taking opioids. Simply put, CPRPs work.

Turk (2002) found in his review of the research studies on such programs that patients have on average a 30% *reduction* in pain following their participation in a CPRP. Remember, this reduction is what patients achieve after they participate in a program that includes tapering opioids. Again, CPRPs work.

Get support from your healthcare provider

We earlier discussed the importance of talking with your prescribing provider about your decision to taper from opioid management and instead learn to self-manage pain. There may be health factors you need to take into account when deciding whether, when and how you taper, and only your own healthcare provider will know them.

Moreover, it's important to talk with your prescribing provider about tapering opioids because you need his or her support to achieve your goal of tapering. You might be surprised by this recommendation. Wouldn't all healthcare providers want patients to be off opioids? In theory, maybe, but in actual practice, many healthcare providers might not support your decision or know how to support it. In my experience, the majority of healthcare providers who feel this way are those who practice in pain clinics that provide long-term opioid management. This statement too might be surprising.

It might be helpful here to explicitly state something that has only been implied in this book up until now. *It's that not all pain clinics are alike.* It's common for patients to not fully understand the differences between pain clinics.

By most conventional standards, there are three types of pain clinics: clinics that focus on surgical procedures; clinics that focus on interventional procedures and long-term opioid management; and clinics that focus on chronic pain rehabilitation.

The first type of practice is largely associated with an acute medical model of care, focusing on spine surgeries. While surgeries on the spine have been done for about a century, it has only been in the last forty years or so that they've been routinely performed for the sole purpose of pain management (Knoeller & Seifried, 2000; McDonnell, 2004). Typical spine surgeries are laminectomies, discectomies, and fusions. Spine surgeons typically have their own clinics, but sometimes they have interventional pain physicians within their group. Either way, these types of pain clinics will typically prescribe opioids, but only while their patients are obtaining procedures. If patients express needs for continued opioid management after they are no longer candidates for more procedures, the providers in these types of clinics will typically refer patients to a pain clinic that provides long-term opioid management.

Long-term opioid management clinics are the second kind of pain clinic. While various types of providers can run this type of clinic, interventional pain physicians commonly head them up. Interventional pain management is "the newest kid on the block," as it were, coming to be quite common in the 1990s. Interventional pain physicians are typically anesthesiologists who have received added training in a variety of interventional pain management procedures, including epidural steroid injections, different types of anesthetic blocks, neuroablation procedures, and implantable pain control devices, such as spinal cord stimulators and intrathecal drug delivery devices. Providers in this second type of clinic typically take over the management of opioid medications and will do so indefinitely, as long as patients don't abuse the medication or require doses that are above the conventional upper limits because of tolerance. While maintaining patients on opioids, they will usually recommend a series of interventional procedures, coupled with physical therapy, and at least a psychological evaluation, if not some type of ongoing follow-up with a psychologist. After completing these therapies, patients are typically maintained on opioids indefinitely, or until they become too tolerant of the medications. When the latter occurs, they refer patients to chronic pain rehabilitation clinics, the third type of conventional pain clinic.

Providers in either surgery clinics or long-term opioid management clinics typically don't taper opioids when patients continue to have chronic pain. Surgeons and interventional pain physicians will taper their patients following a procedure when the procedure is effective in reducing pain. As described above, they pursue a need-based taper in these cases – the patient no longer has pain because the procedure was effective and so the patient no longer needs the medications. All is well. When the procedure doesn't work so well, however, surgeons will typically refer their patients elsewhere to continue the opioids, rather than try to taper a patient who continues to have pain. Interventional pain physicians who provide long-term opioid management will take these patients on and only taper them if the patients are found to be abusing the medications. Typically, the providers in either type of clinic don't have experience in tapering patients who continue to have pain and who aren't abusing the medications, like you.

As such, providers in these clinics often don't know how to support a patient through the process of tapering opioids and learning to self-manage pain. Sometimes, the providers themselves don't think it is possible. Those who prescribe opioids on a long-term basis often think that the use of opioids is essential for proper pain management. I have frequently had patients say to me over the years that they were told by their providers at one of these types of clinics that they will need to be on opioids for the rest of their life, as if opioids were the equivalent of insulin for a diabetic. The problem with this statement is, of course, that opioids aren't like insulin. As we've said, you simply can't expect that opioids will remain effective for the rest of your life, assuming a normal life span. Providers who practice long-term opioid therapies tend to overlook this fact and continue to think that the use of opioids is essential, despite the available evidence.

It's important, then, to find healthcare providers who recognize that it's possible to self-manage pain well without opioids. Indeed, it's important to seek care from providers who recognize that, it's not only possible but necessary if you have a normal life span yet to live. Find healthcare providers who think long-term, because you have a long-term condition. Find healthcare providers who will help you develop a long-term pain management strategy, which truly takes into account the long-term nature of your chronic pain. Find healthcare providers who are experts in guiding you and coaching you to self-manage chronic pain, including how to successfully taper from the long-term use of opioids. You'll find them in CPRPs.

Chapter Summary

You have come to accept that it's in your best interest to learn to self-manage pain and taper from long-term opioid management. It's important to discuss your decision with your prescribing provider and your CPRP providers. There may be important factors about you and your health history, which only they can take into account when coming up with a plan to taper opioids. When pursuing an opioid taper, it's important that you don't abruptly stop their use. Instead, in conjunction with your CPRP providers, develop a plan to taper on a time-scheduled basis. Let intervals of time be your guide as to when to make reductions in the use of the medications. Tapering opioids is a therapy in and of itself because it provides you with real-life opportunities to practice what you've been learning in your CPRP. As such, it's an exposure-based therapy that leads to improved coping. It also leads to empowerment and increased self-confidence. Patients are commonly concerned and apprehensive about tapering opioids. It's easy to catastrophize what it will be like to cope with pain without opioids. However, patients tend to have less pain following the completion of a CPRP. This average reduction occurs even after tapering opioids. Lastly, prior to taking on the task of tapering opioids, it's important to get the support of your prescribing providers, make sure they understand that it's possible to manage pain well without opioids, and that they know how to guide you and coach you. Ordinarily, where you find providers who fit this description is in CPRPs.

CHAPTER TEN

Disability and Returning to Work

We've discussed a number of sensitive topics in this book. We've reviewed and clarified issues related to acceptance, anxiety and depression, and the long-term use of opioids. No treatment manual for a CPRP would be complete without another topic, which is also sensitive to discuss: returning to work.

Chronic pain is a significant factor that leads patients to apply for disability pensions (Andersson, 1999). Many patients with chronic pain apply through their employer's disability policy or through a government program, such as the Social Security Administration in the United States. Some patients are accepted. Many are not.

Indeed, it's difficult to get formal disability benefits for chronic pain. Every day, patients are denied disability benefits or remain in a protracted legal battle to obtain such benefits. They often struggle to understand why it's so difficult. It seems obvious that chronic pain should meet the criteria for a disability. However, their actual difficulty in getting disability for chronic pain suggests that it's not so obvious.

This difference between what actually constitutes a disability and what patients commonly believe should constitute a disability highlights some important distinctions that we should discuss before we get much further into this chapter.

In our healthcare system, the term *disability* is a bit slippery, being used in many different ways by organizations administering disability benefits, by providers, and by patients themselves. Let's discuss these different uses.

Let's begin by discussing the definitions that the Social Security Administration and private disability insurance companies use. These institutions have formal definitions or criteria, which must be met before a patient is provided disability benefits. It's understandable that they need criteria to determine when someone is disabled or not. No one would argue, for instance, that people should get disability just because they feel like it. Rather, they must meet formal criteria for what it means to be disabled in order to get disability benefits. The Social Security Administration maintains a list of criteria for various types of conditions, sometimes referred to as "the Listing" (Social Security Online, 2011). In terms of chronic back pain, for instance, the criteria are a substantial loss of the ability to use a part of the body, like a limb, due to impingement of a nerve that is itself due to either degenerative changes of the spine or a failed spine surgery.

We might notice a few things here. The criteria specify an underlying condition that doesn't refer to how much pain someone has. At first light, this omission might be surprising. Why is there no mention of how much pain you are in? We might presume the reason is that criteria for disability must be based on observable conditions. Pain is inherently a subjective experience. I can't feel or see your pain and you can't feel or see mine. People charged with determining who is disabled or not are in the same boat. How could they really tell how much pain you or anyone else has? They can't. So, the criteria for disability have to be observable by other people, like the people determining whether a patient is disabled or not. Another possible reason is that, as we'll see, a large percentage of people with chronic pain continue to work. What is the difference between their pain and the pain of those who say they're disabled? How could disability examiners tell the difference? They really couldn't. So, again, disability determiners need objective or observable criteria. The solution is to base it on the loss of ability to move a limb, for example, due to nerve impingement that comes from either degenerative changes of the spine or a failed spine surgery. Theoretically, this type of nerve impingement is observable through, for example, an MRI scan. As such, the criteria used by Social Security Disability make some headway in specifying observable criteria.

Nonetheless, the criteria are not fully immune to the problem of how to know when someone meets them or not. Let's look at what the issue is. An underlying condition such as nerve root impingement due to degenerative changes of the spine or a failed back surgery is something observable. Nerve root impingement is often observable, as we said, on an MRI scan. So, we should be able to know when a patient meets that part of the criteria easily enough. However, the substantial loss of function of a body part due to the nerve impingement is not so readily observable. How substantial of a problem does it have to be? For example, a patient can have a condition called 'foot drop' in which the patient lightly drags a foot while walking. The nerves and muscles just don't work right anymore. This condition is typically quite observable. However, patients with foot drop can often still walk and in fact choose to walk, not seeing it as big enough of a problem to use a wheelchair, for example, in their daily lives. Is that a substantial enough problem to meet the criteria for disability? How do you judge when it is a big enough problem and when it isn't? There is some grey area here, isn't there? Let's take it a step further.

Many times, when patients report that they can't do things, the reported loss of function isn't readily observable at all. Would you consider patients disabled if they can still fully use their arms and legs and can in fact walk and stand, but assert that they can't because of pain? Upon inquiry, they acknowledge that they can use their arms and legs. They acknowledge that they can sit, stand and walk. What they assert, however, is that it hurts too much to do one or more of these activities for very long. So, they assert that they can't do these things. Does this scenario count as a substantial loss of functioning?

Organizations charged with administering disability benefits often determine that they aren't disabled. Patients maintain, however, they are disabled. Providers are often somewhere in the middle.

The central question is whether pain by itself causes a loss of function. Organizations charged with administering disability benefits, like the Social Security Administration, typically deny that pain causes the loss of function. It's not part of their definition. As indicated, they define the loss of function with objective criteria – a condition that causes the nerves and muscles to no longer work in the usual ways, leading to an inability to move. Typically, patients acknowledge that their nerves and muscles work right, in terms of being able to move or sit or stand or walk. They allow that their nerves and muscles still work and as such they're physically able to do these things. What they can't do is these things because the pain becomes too intolerable when they do them. The claim is that pain itself causes a loss of function. It's an altogether different understanding of what "loss of function" means. Therein lies the problem.

It's this difference that is so contested in disability applications for chronic pain. The typical outcome for chronic pain patients applying for disability is denial of the application. At best, such as with the Social Security Administration, patients get denied initially and they appeal, which again is denied. Then, with the assistance of a lawyer, they appeal again to get a hearing from a local judge who decides upon their second appeal. Commonly, patients are still denied. The whole affair can take a few years.

We might argue all day long as to whether it should be this way or not. At the end of the day, though, this is basically how it is. Getting disability for chronic pain is difficult for just these reasons: the loss of function which most chronic pain patients state they have is not the same type of loss of function that the criteria for disability requires. This is the current state of affairs when it comes to disability and chronic pain. Again, you might argue that it shouldn't be this way, but it's pretty much this way.

Now, what we can do is the following: let's review an important point that we just made in the above discussion. Let's look at it closely. If you can come to understand and accept it, it holds the key to learning how to become more active, less disabled, and ultimately go back to work. That's right. If you can come to understand this point and accept it, it opens up a whole new way of thinking about your abilities and it becomes clear how you can go back to work.

The key to going back to work

Here's the important point: we said that the disability that most chronic pain patients say they have is based on their inability to cope with the pain if they stand or walk for a period of time or when engaging in chores or returning to work. This loss of function isn't based on their nerves and muscles being unable to move in certain ways, as the nerves and muscles of most pain patients still work. Rather, the loss of function is based on an inability to tolerate the pain when doing these activities. If you buy this distinction, then we can understand and acknowledge that disability, when it comes to most cases of chronic pain, isn't based on an inability to move and do things, but on an inability to sufficiently cope with the pain when moving and doing things.

Why is this important? If an inability to sufficiently cope with pain is the basis of disability, then disability can be overcome because coping with pain can be learned. Unlike someone with paralysis whose nerves and muscles no longer work, your nerves and muscles still work. What you need to do is to learn how to tolerate the pain when you work them. It's possible! The way you do it, of course, is through the two prongs of chronic pain rehabilitation: lifestyle changes that reduce the central sensitization of your nervous system and increasing your abilities to cope with the pain that remains.

It takes strength to accept the notion that it's not pain that leads to disability but rather the difficulty coping with pain. Initially, patients often deny the truth of this statement. Sometimes, they are offended. Don't, however, buy into such stigma. There is nothing morally wrong with you if you struggle to cope with chronic pain. It's okay to admit it. In fact, it's a sign of strength to acknowledge it. It's a sign that you're open to feedback and learning. And it leads to hope – a realistic hope. When you accept it, it becomes the key to taking back control of your life, including returning to work.

In the remainder of this chapter, we'll review how disability is a problem that results from difficulties in coping with pain. From this discussion, we'll see how you can use your CPRP to learn to cope better with pain and thereby return to work. We'll also see why CPRPs are the most successful treatment approach for returning patients back to work. Lastly, we'll discuss why it's important to return to work.

Development of disability in chronic pain is predominantly a self-management problem

We tend to think that pain is what leads to disability. After all, that's what patients say. They can't work because of the pain. Were it not for the pain, they would have remained at work. It seems like a no-brainer.

It seems a no-brainer until we consider how often people with chronic pain become disabled. It's not what you might think. It's not, for instance, that most people with chronic pain are disabled. Rather, it's the opposite. Most people with chronic pain continue to work. This fact remains true even among people whose chronic pain is severe. Numerous studies show that, among people who rate their pain as severe, more than half remain at work (Cassidy, Carroll, & Cote, 1998; Cote, Cassidy, & Carroll, 1998; Linton & Buer, 1995; Von Korff, Dworkin, and La Resche, 1990). So, in determining what leads people to become disabled, there must be more to it than just how much pain they have. Something else must be tipping the scale, in addition to pain, which leads some people to consider themselves to be disabled.

Here is the issue that we've been talking about – difficult to accept, but helpful if you do: it's not the pain, but rather what you go on to do about it that determines whether you become disabled or not.

Research consistently reveals that it's the degree of coping that leads to disability and not pain itself. Fear-avoidance is commonly found to be more disabling than pain (Crombez, Vlaeyen, Heuts, & Lysens, 1999; Denison, Asenlof, & Lindberg, 2004; Vlaeyen & Linton, 2000; Waddell, Newton, Henderson, Somerville, & Main, 1993). As you may recall, fear-avoidance is reacting to pain with alarm and distress and attempting to deal with pain by avoiding activities that are associated with pain. Emotional distress in general has also been found to be a more important factor than pain (Gatchel, Polatin, & Mayer, 1995; Hall, et al., 2011; Wegener, Castillo, Haythornwaite, MacKenzie, & Bosse, 2011). Catastrophizing, too, is more important than pain when it comes to who becomes disabled (Sullivan, Lynch, & Clark, 2005; Sullivan, Stanish, Waite, Sullivan, & Tripp, 1998). Other stressors, such as legal conflicts, socioeconomic problems, and other psychological problems have all been found to be more important than pain itself (Andersson, 1999; Gatchel, Polatin, & Mayer, 1995; Turner, Jensen, & Romano, 2000). All these non-pain-related factors can tip the scale. They can make coping with pain so problematic that people come to conclude that they can't function with the pain. The issue, then, is that it's not just pain. It's in how you're reacting to the pain.

Some readers wonder whether the severity of injury plays a role in who becomes disabled. The research shows that it has little role in determining who continues to work and who doesn't. When comparing subjective responses to pain, such as fear-avoidance, with objective findings, such as MRI findings, coping continues to play a much greater role in disability (Boos, et al., 2000; Carragee, Alamin, Miller, & Carragee, 2005).

These findings echo what you see in the clinic. Patients with severe health problems commonly continue to work and patients with little to no objective findings often don't work. This fact reflects what we learned about degenerative disc disease in Chapter Seven: many people have degenerative changes without any pain and some people have pain without any degenerative changes. That is to say, the relationship between the severity of degenerative changes of the spine and pain is minimal. So again, it's not so much the health problem that leads to disability, but how you respond to the problem.

Despite any initial surprise, it stands to reason that disability when it comes to chronic pain is at heart a coping problem. People who cope well with adversity tend to continue to function well. Those who don't cope so well tend to struggle. Let's return to our pain and coping spectrum illustration:

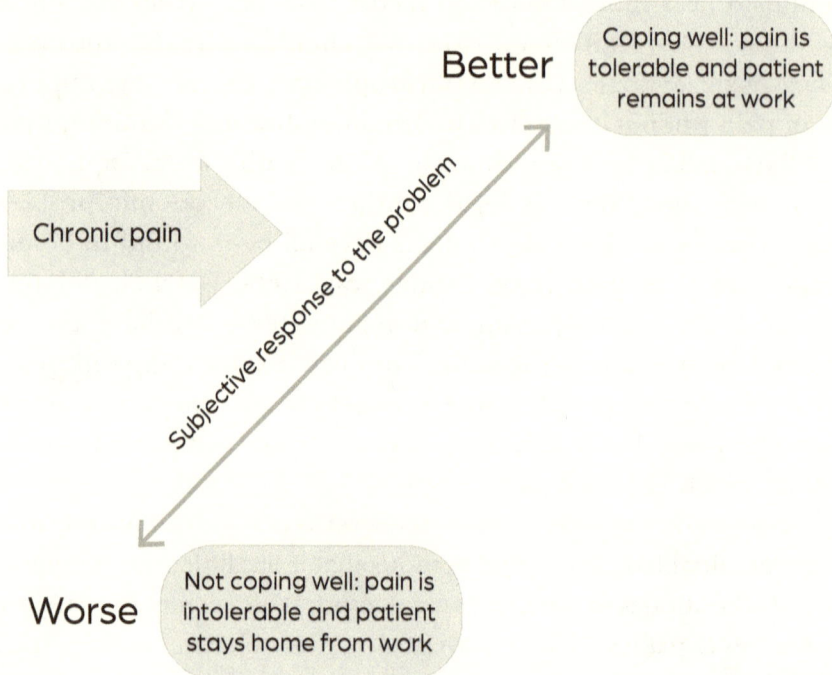

People who cope well with pain tend to remain focused on the activities of life, like work and social or recreational activities. They maintain a sense of well-being by accepting the chronicity of their pain, refraining from illness behaviors, and remaining focused on pursuing the activities of life. People who don't cope so well tend to become alarmed by pain, refrain from accepting it, engage in illness behaviors, and become fear-avoidant. Their overall responses to chronic pain lead to emotional distress and functional impairment. In other words, they come to see themselves as disabled.

Now, here again, when making such observations, we don't judge patients who are disabled. We don't buy into such stigma. We talk about the importance of coping without judgment in other areas of life. Drill sergeants don't expect new recruits to know how to cope with the adversities of war and then judge them when the recruits don't know how. Rather, they simply assume, without judgment, that the recruits don't know how to cope and so have them go through boot camp – an extensive training that shows them how to physically and emotionally cope with adversity. By doing so, the recruits move up the coping spectrum, becoming better able to deal with the problems they might face in war. It's what boot camp is for. There is no sensitivity about it.

Similarly, it's okay to acknowledge that you can get better at coping with chronic pain. No matter where you are on the coping spectrum, you can always get better at coping. It takes coaching and practice, but most importantly, an openness to learning. To be open, though, you have to get past the stigma. You have to get over the sensitivity of acknowledging that functioning in life with chronic pain, like going back to work, is really about getting better at coping. There's no shame in needing to learn how to cope better. Just like soldiers learning how to cope in boot camp, chronic pain patients learn how to cope in CPRPs. Patients learn how every day and you can too.

In fact, when you accept the notion of how important coping is, you open up a whole new way of getting better and returning to work. Indeed, there is simply no end to getting better at changing your subjective reactions to pain. Patients can get so good at remaining grounded in the presence of pain that the pain becomes like white noise. It's like a fan that remains on in the room, but which only occasionally catches their attention. Most of the time, they are engaging in the activities of their life.

Learning to cope better with chronic pain and going back to work are also important because there are significant problems that can occur when disabled. This observation too is a sensitive topic, but let's talk a little about these problems.

Problems associated with long-term disability

When discussing problems associated with disability, it's important that we initially take note that it's a good thing that we have a disability system. Whether it's through the Social Security Administration or private disability insurers, it's important to have a back-up when health adversities strike. No one should lose everything and become homeless because they're injured or ill and unable to earn a livelihood. The disability system serves a necessary and essential service for our society.

At the same time, however, there are some downsides to it. Work gives us more than just a paycheck. It structures our daily lives. Without regular work, each day becomes the same day, day after day, without any purpose or focus. Work also structures our sleep-wake cycle, so that we are awake during the day and asleep at night. Without regular work, we can often come to sleep at irregular times throughout the 24-hour cycle. We can subsequently experience social isolation and depression.

Work gives us a focus for our attention, time, and energy. Without it, we can come to focus too much on the problems of life, like chronic pain. Sitting around the house with nothing to do leads to a persistent focus on pain, which itself leads to a persistent sense of alarm. From here, it's easy to spiral downward, becoming focused on what you've lost, what you can't do, how alone and misunderstood you feel, how depressed you are, and how anxious or hopeless the future seems.

Regular work also gives us a sense of friendship and community. We spend a lot of time with our coworkers. We get to know them and like them and they like us. Even if we don't become close friends with them, we still have a sense of common purpose and camaraderie with our coworkers. In these ways, work keeps us in touch with the outside world. These things can fall by the wayside when not working on a regular basis. We can subsequently become lonely and chronically bored.

Work also gives us an identity and role in the family. We often identify ourselves with what we do – "I'm a police officer" or "I'm a contractor." We take pride in who we are and what we do. Without regular work, we lose this sense of identity and source of self-esteem. We can also lose our role as a provider in the family, which also wears on our self-esteem.

Work also gives us a sense of purpose or progress in our lives. Whether we're talking about getting additional training over the years or moving up the hierarchy of an organization or moving up the pay grade, work gives us a feeling of progress. We feel like we are going somewhere in life. Without regular work, it's hard to maintain this sense of progress in life. Patients sometimes ask me, "What's the point of it all?" or "Why am I here?" They struggle to find an answer. Work can provide that answer.

Without work, it is hard to cope with life's problems, including chronic pain. How do you cope well with adversity when you lack structure to your day, lack a focus for your attention, lack community, lack a sense of productivity, lack self-esteem, and when you feel like you are going nowhere? The answer, of course, is that it is really hard.

This point brings us to another tenet of chronic pain rehabilitation: *returning to work is not something you do as a result of getting better; it's one of the ways that you are going to get better.* This tenet stands the acute medical model of care on its head. In the acute medical model, you wait for a healthcare specialist to fix your condition, remain off work and stay home, take medicines, and once you obtain your cure, you get better and then, and only then, return to work. In the rehabilitation model of care, you accept the chronicity of your health condition and you seek healthcare specialists to coach you on returning to work despite your condition. You practice self-managing your health while returning to work and over time you get better at it.

The rehabilitation approach of returning to work despite your health condition leads to increased coping. If you have been off work for some time, you likely have begun to experience the problems we described above. However, when you practice self-managing pain and come to see that you're doing more, you can take the next step of returning to work in some capacity. In turn, returning to work leads to increased coping because you again have a structure for your daily life; you have a focus for your attention; you have a sense of productivity and self-esteem again; you have community; and you have a sense of meaning and purpose to your life again. All these benefits subsequently make you more able to cope with pain. Thus, learning how to return to work is a way that you get better – not what you do as a result of getting better.

In the introduction of this book, I described individuals who self-manage pain so well that while chronic pain continues in their life, it causes no significant problems in their life. It causes no significant emotional distress or sense of disability. When asked about their lives, they talk about their work, their family, hobbies, and activities. It might not even occur to them to talk about their chronic pain. I asked you, "What would it be like to put chronic pain into the background of your life like that?"

Everything in this book has been leading you to this point. By learning how to self-manage pain, you come to find that you can live well despite having chronic pain.

Chronic pain rehabilitation is an exposure-based therapy that leads to returning to work

CPRPs are set up on a daily basis for three to four weeks for a reason. It simulates going back to work. When you participate in a CPRP, you commit to engaging in therapeutic activities every day. At first, you might not be able to do everything. However, you're at least showing up and trying. The staff coach and support you. As you keep trying, you get better at it. You are, of course, learning how to self-manage pain, which is the focus of CPRPs. At the same time, however, you're also keeping a daily schedule of activities outside the home. A budding sense of confidence takes hold. You're doing something that looks a lot like work. After three or four weeks, you come to realize that you can in fact return to many types of work, because you're already doing it. You're keeping what amounts to a schedule of flexible, light duty activities on a daily basis outside the home over the course of a number of weeks.

CPRPs are thus an exposure-based therapy that shows you how to return to work and regain the confidence that you can in fact do it. We've discussed the nature of CPRPs as an exposure-based therapy before, in the section on tapering opioid medications. Now, we see that it's also an exposure-based therapy for returning to work.

Chronic pain rehabilitation programs generalize to real work

Sometimes, patients have a position waiting for them upon completion of a CPRP. For instance, they've been on short-term disability or a temporary medical leave from their job. In such cases, patients commonly return to their position because they've come to see how they can keep a full-time schedule of daily activities for weeks – all the while self-managing their pain at a tolerable level. Other times, patients return to their position on a gradual basis, starting out on a part-time basis and increasing their hours according to some agreed-upon schedule until they're back at work full-time. Patients routinely succeed in doing so because they've learned how and have had the time to practice before actually returning to work – all in their CPRP.

Still other times, patients have been on long-term disability or have been off work for some time and so have no actual position to which they can return. In these cases, upon their completion of the program, they begin looking for work. The CPRP staff coaches them how to handle interview questions, such as why they haven't been working for so long or whether they have any limitations.

In the meantime, however, it's standard for CPRP staff to recommend that the patient begin volunteering part-time. It doesn't matter where someone volunteers – that's up to them and their interests and values. What matters is that they transfer their newly learned skills for remaining active in a work environment. Volunteering is work – just not for pay. Like work, it has all the same benefits that we described above, other than a paycheck. It gets you out of the house on a regular basis and it structures your day, giving you a reason to get up in the morning. You engage in a meaningful and productive activity that provides you with a focus for your attention and a source of self-esteem. You are involved with a group of people outside your immediate family, which provides you with camaraderie and a sense of community. But it also gives you more.

Just as importantly, volunteering provides you with an opportunity to demonstrate a recent work history. You transfer your newly learned abilities to maintain a daily schedule to your volunteer job and in this position, you practice maintaining your schedule. You come to know how to self-manage pain so well that you show up for work even on bad pain days. As such, you prove to yourself that you can be accountable to an organization. Moreover, you now have a work history that demonstrates to a potential employer that you can be accountable!

It all starts, however, with your participation in a CPRP that teaches you how to be active on a daily basis and regain the confidence that you really can do so.

CPRPs are powerful interventions. The research is consistent. There is simply no better chronic pain treatment than CPRPs when it comes to returning to work. Patients return to work at a rate of 40-60% following participation in a CPRP. This statistic is all the more remarkable when you find out that the average patient who participates in a CPRP has been off work for seven years (Turk, 2002). Again, when compared to any other treatment for chronic pain, CPRPs are the most effective in helping patients to return to work. Now, you can see why.

Chapter Summary

Disability is a sensitive topic. Patients often have strong feelings about it. Many chronic pain patients see themselves as disabled and yet only some of them get disability. Organizations charged with administering disability benefits, such as the Social Security Administration, typically don't define chronic pain as sufficient to meet the criteria for disability. There needs to be an observable failure of the nerves and muscles to work right. Patients often assert that they nonetheless can't do things, even if their nerves and muscles still work right. They report that the loss of function is due to pain. The difference between these causes of disability is often what leads chronic pain patients to get denied disability benefits. Most organizations charged with administering disability benefits simply do not see an inability to tolerate pain when doing the activities of life as enough to meet the criteria for disability. This discussion of problems associated with trying to get disability leads to an important insight. Patients perceive themselves as disabled because they're unable to tolerate the pain when doing activities of life, like work. If you accept this position, then the disability that patients state they have can be overcome. It's a process of learning to self-manage pain. CPRPs are designed to teach patients how to cope with pain and to do so while becoming more active. In fact, the daily schedule exposes patients to a schedule of activities that is similar to work and the team of expert providers teaches patients how to cope with pain while maintaining a high level of daily activities. Patients consequently learn how to keep a daily schedule of activities, which is similar to work. Just as importantly, over the extended period of time that they are in a program, patients regain the confidence that they can in fact do it. They learn how to go back to work and that they can go back to work. Overcoming disability and returning to work is possible. Patients do it every day in CPRPs.

CHAPTER ELEVEN

How to Respond to Pain Flares and Other Advanced Coping Skills

By this point in the program, you've made various healthy lifestyle changes and you're changing how you subjectively react to pain. You practice these things on a daily basis. Sometimes, you are successful. Sometimes, you are not. Sometimes, you forget to do them, but you later remember and start up again. The goal isn't perfection, but just to try and keep trying. As long as you practice making these changes, you'll get better at them. The two prongs of self-management are skills like any other set of skills and the more you practice, the better you'll get at them. And the better you get at self-managing pain, the more your overall well-being improves.

Let's move on to advanced coping skills. In doing so, we build on a few things that you know by now. One, we build on our understanding of the two prongs of self-management – reducing central sensitization through lifestyle changes and increasing your ability to cope with pain. Two, we build on the insight that we had in Chapter Seven. Namely, when it comes to coping, how you make sense of your pain matters. It matters how you go on to respond to pain. In this chapter, we'll review a new way for you to make sense of how and why pain flares occur. From this new understanding, you'll know how to more effectively react to the flare itself.

How to make sense of a pain flare

Suppose you wake up today and it's clear that it's going to be a bad pain day. In such a scenario, what initially comes to mind? If you're like most patients, you think one of four things.

One, you might ask yourself, "What did I do yesterday?" and go on to think of any activities that might have aggravated your chronic pain condition. In other words, you make sense of the pain flare in terms of potential activities that might have irritated the original injury that started your pain. For example, you think that you did too much yesterday and you irritated the degenerative changes in your spine. As a result, you have more pain today.

Two, you might think that it must be the weather. Maybe, it's raining or it's cold outside. As such, you think that the increased pain is due to the weather. The underlying assumption is that changes in the weather affect the original injury or illness that started the pain. You think, for instance, that the cold front is affecting your osteoarthritis.

Three, you might come to think that the increased pain is because the original injury or illness is getting worse. You think, for instance, that the degenerative changes in your spine are progressively degenerating.

Four, you don't know why you have increased pain. You consider it for a while, but you can't seem to identify what's aggravating the original injury or illness. Despite being at a loss as to why your pain is worse today, you still assume that something must be aggravating the original health condition that started the pain.

In brief, patients tend to think that pain flares occur because something is aggravating the condition that caused the pain in the first place. Like activity, weather, or deteriorating health, something must have aggravated the original injury or illness. This way of making sense of a pain flare matters.

If you think that pain flares are the result of something aggravating the original injury or illness, then the natural reaction is to stop aggravating it. Whether it's chronic low back pain that started with a lifting injury or diabetic neuropathy in your feet, if you have a bad pain day and you conceptualize it as the result of something aggravating your back or feet, the reaction to your increased pain is to stop using your back or feet.

If you think it's physical activity, you will stop doing it. If you think it's the weather, you'll stay inside at home. If you think it's deteriorating health, you'll tend to rest. In other words, in all these cases, you're going to stay home, rest and become inactive. Moreover, you're likely going to feel vulnerable and helpless because, with the exception of physical activity, the perceived causes are all things outside your control.

Notice what happens, then, when you make sense of a pain flare as something that is aggravating your original injury or condition: you end up doing exactly what we know leads to poor coping and more pain: illness behaviors, avoidance of activities, and increased emotional distress.

More often than not, it's a mistake to think that a pain flare is the result of something that is aggravating the original injury or illness. It's a mistake because pragmatically it leads to poor coping responses to the pain flare. It's also a mistake because this way of thinking about a pain flare is most often inaccurate.

Change the way you make sense of a pain flare

There are two other reasons for pain flares, which you should always take into account. They are how dysregulated your nervous system is and how well you're coping at the time of the flare. Let's take one at a time.

How stressed is my nervous system?

We have learned that, as a chronic pain patient, you have something more than simply a long-lasting injury or illness that has failed to heal. You have a complicated chronic pain syndrome. What initially started your pain (i.e., the initial injury or illness) isn't now the only thing that is maintaining your pain on a chronic course. Specifically, because of multiple biological and psychological stressors, your nervous system has become stuck in a persistent state of reactivity that is called *central sensitization*. It is central sensitization that is now the main cause of your chronic pain.

We can apply this understanding of central sensitization to how you should respond to pain flares. Specifically, if you experience a pain flare and subsequently search for what might be aggravating the injury or illness that initially started your pain, then, more often than not, you're looking in the wrong place. Instead, look to what might be exacerbating your central sensitization.

What might exacerbate central sensitization? Let's quickly review where central sensitization comes from. Central sensitization develops as a result of the stress response to both pain and other stressors that occur because of the pain. Pain and these stressors make the nervous system more reactive and the increased reactivity of the nervous system further increases pain. So, what might make this condition worse and thus cause more pain? The answer is stress.

The first question that any chronic pain patient should ask when experiencing a pain flare is what else in life is going on that is causing stress to the nervous system. Stress is the most likely culprit for pain flares.

There are any number of stressors that are common to living with chronic pain: insomnia; relationship conflicts; work problems and financial stressors; anxiety and depression; lack of structure and focus for your day; loss of self-esteem; loss of your role in the family; and so on. All of these problems cause stress, which in turn elicits the stress response. The stress response increases reactivity of the nervous system and such reactivity increases pain.

How common is it to have such stressors? It's very common. It's so common that the stress of these problems can no longer be obvious when they occur. It can become so familiar that it tends to go unnoticed. As such, when pain flares occur, the stress that has led to the increased pain isn't always immediately apparent. Patients subsequently tend to look elsewhere, such as to activities they may have done yesterday or to the weather, to explain the flare.

Now, I'm not saying that activities or the weather never cause pain flares. However, it's about getting the proportions right. When experiencing a pain flare, it's more productive to look to what is stressing your nervous system and attempt to resolve the effects of the stress than to look to what must have aggravated the underlying condition that started the pain in the first place. This way of responding goes hand in hand with accepting the nature of your chronic pain. You have chronic pain, not a long-lasting injury that has failed to heal. It's more accurate and effective to respond to a pain flare by attempting to down-regulate your nervous system than stopping your physical activities, avoiding the weather, or avoiding whatever else you think might be aggravating your original injury or health condition.

As we've noted, such responses are what people who cope well with pain do. Now you know why.

The upshot of this discussion is the following: when experiencing a pain flare, don't look to what might be aggravating the original condition that started your pain and don't engage in illness behaviors as a consequence of conceptualizing the flare in this way. Rather, look to the main problem that you have now, which is central sensitization, and what might be exacerbating it. The first question to ask yourself is "What's the condition of my nervous system and what might be aggravating it?" It will likely be some type of stress. Then, take actions to reduce the reactivity of your nervous system.

How well have I been coping lately?

The second question to ask yourself when experiencing a pain flare is "How well have I been coping lately?" In other words, you can come at the problem of what causes a pain flare from the perspective of the subjective experience of coping.

Give consideration to your overall well-being – how you've been thinking and feeling – prior to the pain flare and during it. Reflect on what occurred prior to the flare and think about how you reacted. Likely some stressful event occurred and you had some cognitive (i.e., thinking) and emotional (i.e., feelings) reaction to it.

Upon such reflection, suppose you find that you've been irritable lately. You've been impatient with the kids and your spouse has been bugging you in ways she usually doesn't. As such, you come to see that it's been in this context that your headaches are more intense today. Or suppose you recognize that your depression is worsening; you see that you've been more tearful lately and everything seems more of a struggle. You come to see the correspondence of your worsening mood and your increasing back pain.

Sometimes it's helpful to see your overt behaviors as a clue to your internal coping. Health behaviors, specifically, are often an indicator of how well or how poorly we're coping. Suppose, upon self-reflection, you observe that you've had a big bowl of ice cream most every night in the last few weeks and from this recognition you see that everything has seemed such a struggle lately; you subsequently make the connection that you've been more depressed lately and maybe that's why your back hurts more. Notice that the overt health behavior of stress-eating clued you into the current state of your overall well-being and subsequently why you had the pain flare. Any of the common health behaviors may reflect our level of internal coping: besides eating, they are exercising, stress management behaviors, drinking, and smoking. When coping well, we tend to be on top of these behaviors, whereas when not coping well, we tend to let them go. So, if it's hard for you to readily observe your degree of internal coping, look to your health behaviors as potential clues to your well-being.

As you do so, consider the following diagram as a model for how to make sense of a pain flare:

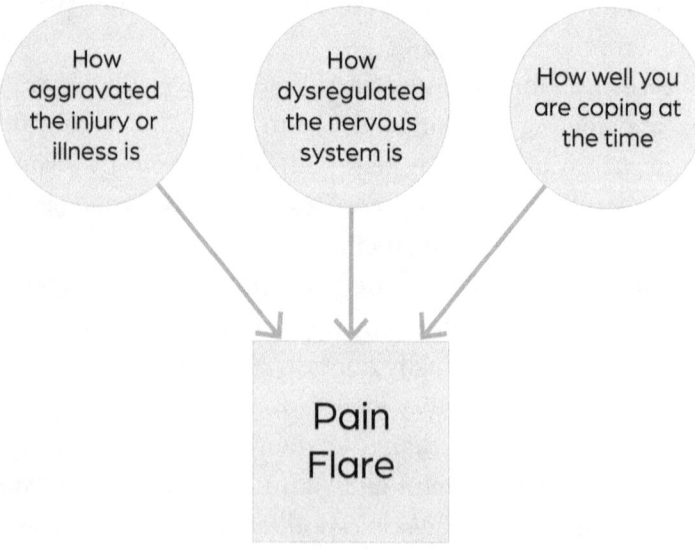

All three factors may have a role. The second and third, though, are likely the most important to keep in mind when considering what is causing a pain flare.

How to respond to a pain flare, now that you understand where it is coming from

You now understand that the current state of your nervous system and your current coping level are what are primarily responsible for the flare. From here, take three further steps to respond effectively to a pain flare: 1) observe your current automatic negative reactions to the flare, 2) challenge their accuracy and come to see that they are untrue, and 3) replace them with more effective coping reactions.

First, observe your present reactions to the flare. Consider your cognitive reactions – how you are thinking about it. Are you catastrophizing? Suppose you observe yourself thinking that the pain flare is evidence of your inevitable decline to becoming wheelchair-bound. Or suppose you find yourself thinking that because of the increased pain you'll never be able to do anything today. Maybe you start thinking that you never get a break. It consequently seems evident that life is always bad. You subsequently take note of the fine line between catastrophization and all-or-nothing thinking. These automatic negative thoughts fly by in a moment and seem obviously true.

Notice too that you have a set of common emotional reactions that occur alongside these automatic negative thoughts. They are fear, anxiety, loss, helplessness, anger, or depression. These emotions can sap the energy right out of you. Once overtaken by them, it's easy to respond with illness behaviors – going back to bed, resting on the couch, sleeping, avoiding activities, and taking more medications.

So, it's important to observe your cognitive and emotional reactions to the flare.

Second, use your observational self to think about and challenge these cognitive and emotional reactions to the pain flare. Ask yourself: how true are they? Develop a sensitivity to hearing yourself use words like "never" and "always" and "I can't" and any other words and phrases that convey a sense of certainty about your pain. Once you hear yourself saying them, try to step out of them and see that their truth is only apparent. Try to recognize that you can still do things even with more pain. You don't "have to" lie down and become inactive. You subsequently recognize that such categorical statements that involve words like "never," "always," "can't" and "have to" are rarely true.

Try to remember that pain flares come and go and rarely, if ever, anything catastrophic happens. Literally think about the times when you've had flares in the past. As a result, you find that catastrophized scenarios rarely ever come true. When you step out of the anxious moment, and look back on the trajectory of your chronic pain and how many times you've had pain flares, you likely won't see a continuous decline. Rather, you see ups and downs. As a result of these considerations, practice reassuring yourself that you know what the pain flare is, you've had them before, and you've gotten through them. Recognize that, actually, you've been getting better at working through them. Literally, tell yourself these things. By challenging your catastrophizations in these ways, you remain less anxious, more grounded, and more able to cope with the flare.

Similarly, challenge any all-or-nothing thinking or I-can't-thinking that you're doing now that you have a pain flare. Try to step out of your either-or thinking and see that there are always more options than being all-in or all-out. Suppose you wake up with a pain flare and your kid has a school concert later in the day. Challenge the seemingly obvious conclusion that you can't go. Instead, consider how you might go, reminding yourself that it's okay to modify how you'll go. It's untrue that you either have to go exactly as you always have in the past or don't go at all. You can get a seat in the back so you can stand if you need to. You can engage in diaphragmatic breathing while listening. You can practice focusing your attention on the video that you take of the concert, rather than the pain. There are all sorts of options besides all-or-nothing. You just have to make an effort to creatively think of them.

Third, once you've observed your reactions and have successfully challenged them, you practice replacing them with what you have learned so far. Consider what we have learned about good coping. What do people who cope well with pain do?

They take steps to relax their nervous system. They engage in extra breathing exercises. They stretch. They make sure they take a walk. They might take an extra hot bath. They also take steps to resolve their stressors. They reach out to their friends and loved ones. They get support for managing their stress. They read books on stress management and practice what they learn.

What they don't do is become alarmed by pain, think that something is aggravating the original injury, and stay home, rest, and take more medications.

Rather, they remind themselves that they know what their pain is – that it's central sensitization and that they are simply having *more of the same*. They don't need to have it checked out and be told that it's more of the same. A good rule of thumb here is that if the pain flare is more of the same, then you don't need to have it evaluated by a healthcare provider. If, however, the pain is a new pain, whether it's in a new location or has a different quality to it, then it's worth having it evaluated. Of course, if you've had a new, acute injury or illness, then it too should be evaluated. But, if the pain flare is the same pain that you've always had, just more of it, then stay grounded and self-manage it.

People who cope with chronic pain well also stay active in the presence of pain. They use the check-engine light metaphor to remind themselves that they shouldn't get alarmed, pull over, and stop driving. Instead, they react to a pain flare by making sure they get out of the house and get involved in something. They go to work. They go to the party. They go to the kid's concert. By doing so, they keep their focus on what's positive in life. They maintain their self-esteem and involvement in life. They relegate chronic pain, even pain flares, to the background of life.

Now that's what good coping looks like: reducing the reactivity of your nervous system; maintaining positive cognitive and emotional reactions to pain; and staying active. They are how you self-manage pain and they are how you self-manage when you have more of the same – otherwise known as a pain flare.

Advanced coping – taking responsibility for chronic pain now that you have it, revisited

Regarding our illustration of the three contributing factors to a pain flare, the astute reader will understand that our discussion of how to make sense of a pain flare also goes for how to make sense of chronic pain in general – whether in a flare or not.

It would be helpful to make explicit something that has been implied up to now in this book. It's the fact that any level of chronic pain – whether at the level of a pain flare or not – is the result of the three contributing factors. The three factors are the present state of the original injury or illness that started the pain, the present state of your centrally sensitized nervous system, and your current level of coping.

Moreover, in most individuals, the latter two are the most important determining factors to the present level of pain. For the conditions commonly seen in CPRPs, the pain levels of patients are mostly a function of how reactive their nervous systems are and how they're coping with pain, and not how their original injury or illness is doing.

How else do we explain the common phenomena of people who have the same condition, and even have the same level of severity of the condition, but have different levels of pain? It's the current state of the nervous system and the current level of coping that determines the levels of chronic pain, not the degree of the original injury or illness.

With some patients, and in certain quarters of the healthcare field, this idea might be construed as heresy. At the very least, it sounds dangerously like blaming the patient.

This perspective, though, misunderstands the point. It confuses stigma with the facts. Let's take a second look at the facts.

The facts pertain to the difference between acute pain and chronic pain. Typically, when we have an acute injury, the pain we experience is the direct result of how severe the injury is. Less severe injuries tend to be less painful and more severe injuries tend to be more painful. This direct relationship between severity of injury and severity of pain isn't true, however, when it comes to chronic pain. Chronic pain is largely the result of central sensitization, not a long-lasting injury. This fact is why people with chronic pain can have intolerable levels of pain in the absence of a severe injury. Indeed, it's the case most of the time. Patients with chronic pain aren't always (or even typically) the most severely injured. It's just not what explains their pain. What does explain it is how centrally sensitized their nervous systems are and how skilled they are in coping with it.

These facts about the psychophysiological states of the patient don't imply blame of the patient. They are as legitimate a way of having a health problem as any other way.

The good news is that these two things – the present state of your nervous system and your present skill level at coping – can change. By learning how to change them, you can get better. You just have to take ownership and responsibility for learning how.

Now, notice that we aren't talking about blame here. We are talking about having an accurate understanding of the facts and taking responsibility for your health and well-being, chronic pain included. You can have responsibility without blame. We don't have to confuse stigma with the facts.

Everything you've been learning in your CPRP has focused on how to self-manage the two factors that largely lead to the chronicity of your pain. The first prong of self-management aims to beneficially modify one factor that leads to how much pain you experience – central sensitization. It really does matter how dysregulated your nervous system is. You've been learning how to pay attention to it and how to reduce its reactivity. The second prong of self-management aims to beneficially modify the second factor that leads to how much pain you experience – how skilled you are at coping with pain. In your CPRP, you've been learning how to pay attention to your old ways of coping, change them, and replace them with better ways of coping. You've overcome any potential stigma for not already being an expert at it and have allowed yourself to be in the student role. You've allowed the CPRP staff to teach you and you've practiced it. You are now getting good at it. There's no shame, and it's your gain.

So, as we come to a close, consider our model of pain levels again, but let's modify it in order to illustrate pain levels in general, and not just pain flares:

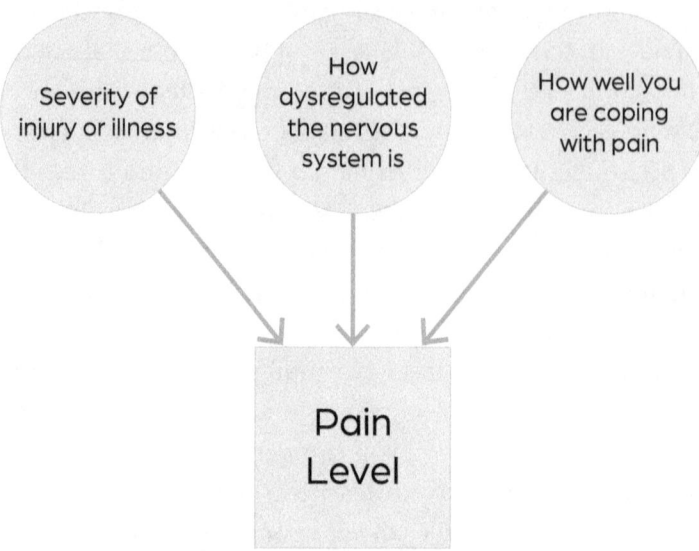

The smaller circle illustrates that the severity of injury or illness is a less important contributor to pain levels than the other factors. Indeed, for many chronic pain patients, the initial injury or illness has long since healed. Even if it hasn't, though, the most important contributing factors to your present level of pain are the current state of your nervous system and how well you are coping at the present time.

As you go forward in life with chronic pain, spend your time and energy on the most important factors – reducing the central sensitization and getting better at coping.

Chapter Summary

Patients commonly think of pain flares as the result of something aggravating the original injury or illness that started their pain in the first place. Common examples that come to mind are physical activities, weather, or evidence of the inevitable decline of one's health. Sometimes, patients are unsure what might be causing the flare, but still assume that something must be aggravating the original condition.

These attributions are typically a mistake. The predominant reasons for pain flares are stress-related exacerbations of central sensitization and difficulties in coping. Numerous stressors occur with chronic pain. Difficulties in coping also commonly occur. It's important to observe stressors and other difficulties in coping, recognize them, and come up with ways to overcome them. We can use this insight into how pain flares occur to explain pain levels in general. What largely determines the levels of pain that chronic pain patients have on any given day are the present level of reactivity of their nervous system and their present level of coping. These are the two most important determining factors to self-manage and they correspond to the two prongs of self-management: lifestyle changes that reduce central sensitization and increasing the abilities to cope with the pain that remains.

CHAPTER TWELVE

Putting It All together and Finding Balance

Let's take stock of the changes you're making. You've been reading this book as a companion to your participation in a CPRP. Alternatively, because of obstacles to obtaining care in a CPRP, you've been reading this book as a companion to treatment with an individual chronic pain rehabilitation provider, or even just as a stand-alone self-help book. In any case, you've been learning and practicing the two prongs of self-management: lifestyle changes which, when done over time, reduce the central sensitization of your nervous system and b) increase your abilities to cope with the pain that remains. By this point, you're actively engaging in both prongs.

An inventory of the changes in the first prong of self-management includes:

- Regular mild, low-impact aerobic exercise
- Daily relaxation therapy
- Stopping pain talk and behaviors
- Regular hot baths or some other, similar, hot water therapy
- Reduced caffeine use
- Reduced nicotine use (or, ideally, stopping altogether)
- Regulating your sleep-wake cycle
- Tapering opioid medication use under the direction of your CPRP providers
- Use of non-narcotic pain medications at the direction of your CPRP providers

By making these lifestyle changes and practicing them over time, you reduce pain by re-regulating your nervous system back down to a more normal level.

An inventory of the second prong of self-management involves these changes:

- Fully accept the chronicity of pain
- Become ready for change and accept responsibility for managing your pain
- Accept that you aren't already an expert in coping with chronic pain and accept being in a student role when it comes to participating in your therapies
- Practice maintaining an observational self
- Learn that your chronic pain is more than just the long-lasting pain of your original injury or illness and that it is predominantly due to central sensitization and your present level of coping
- Begin changing your attitude about opioid medications: that they are more problematic than you've previously thought, that it's possible to manage pain well without opioid medications and that in fact most people with chronic pain do it
- Recognize that tapering opioids is an integral part of the process of learning to cope better with pain and that you overcome your persistent vulnerability to pain when you let go of taking these medications
- Begin work towards overcoming anxiety, including getting psychotherapy if you have an anxiety disorder
- Begin work towards overcoming depression, including getting psychotherapy if depressed
- Practice catching yourself catastrophizing and challenge it
- Practice catching yourself engaging in all-or-nothing thinking and challenge it
- Practice catching yourself engaging in I-can't-thinking and challenge it
- Stop reacting to pain as if its acute pain: turn off the alarm bells and remain grounded in the presence of pain
- Stop engaging in illness behaviors such as resting, staying home, activity avoidance, and taking more medications

- Start reacting to pain as the chronic pain that it is: when in pain, get out of the house and get busy with something, but pace yourself
- Reduce perfectionistic and workaholic characteristics: practice maintaining the attitude that "good is good enough" and pace yourself
- Learn and accept that typically chronic pain isn't inevitably going to get worse: degenerative changes of the spine aren't inevitably degenerative; they often get better; they are common in the general population and are commonly not painful
- Reduce fear of your pain condition and practice having confidence that the human spine isn't fragile; typically, it's a durable piece of equipment that has served the human race well for millennia
- Practice having confidence that normal daily activities don't make degenerative changes of the spine worse and that even accidents, such as slips and falls, don't tend to make such changes worse
- Overcome fear of pain by challenging your tendency to avoid activities of your daily life and gain confidence that you can become active again
- Catch yourself thinking of yourself as a victim and challenge it; observe how you've been taking steps to get better and how it's helping; begin to feel the empowerment and confidence that comes when taking back control of pain
- Be open and learn from the experts: try to do what people who cope well with pain do – in response to chronic pain, they get active, not less active
- Practice relegating pain to the background of your attention, like you might with a broken check-engine light that remains lit on your dashboard
- Return to paid or volunteer work, or some other regular, structured activity, preferably outside the home, because it will help you to cope better

It's striking, isn't it? There are so many ways to self-manage pain. There truly is so much hope when you embrace chronic pain rehabilitation as the way to get better.

Accepting that you are making progress

At the end of their participation in CPRPs, patients commonly ask, "Why didn't anyone ever refer me to this program earlier?" The question comes from the contrast that they see and feel at the time. They have improved so much. They feel less pain, anxiety, and depression. Maybe, they're no longer anxious or depressed at all. They're no longer taking opioids and part of them still can't quite believe it's true. However, the proof is in the pudding. They're managing their pain without opioids and they feel good. What they are feeling is empowered and confident, feelings that they haven't had in a long time.

And yet, they can't help but think of all those years they spent struggling – struggling to find a specialist to fix them, struggling with one failed treatment after another, struggling with providers who kept recommending the same procedures and therapies again and again, struggling with providers to get opioid medications for pain, struggling with hating the fact that they were taking opioids while at the same time believing that they wouldn't be able to live with the pain if they didn't have them.

But, now, here they are feeling good, off their medications, and returning to work or some type of volunteer job. The contrast between then and now is unsettling. And so they ask, "Why didn't anyone ever refer me to this program earlier?"

The answer is complex. There might be various answers to this question, all of which might be true at different times with different patients and with different providers.

One possibility is the acceptance issue. At a certain point in having chronic pain, it's hard to accept that pain is truly chronic. Patients, understandably, look for something that will cure their pain condition. More generally, we also live in a society that doesn't do acceptance very well. On the one hand, we are a can-do society and have made many technological advances across many domains in life. On the other hand, this can-do attitude can lead to a persistent and yet false belief that a fix can be found for all of life's problems. We tend to struggle with accepting that certain problems can't be fixed. As such, when it comes to chronic pain, we seek surgeries and interventional procedures and medications, which appear as if they might be a fix, but aren't in reality. Oftentimes, then, patients have to become ready for participating in a CPRP, as the emphasis on acceptance is tantamount to giving up hope in a cure. So, to the question of why a referral didn't come earlier, the answer may be that the patient wasn't yet ready.

Another possibility is that healthcare providers often fail to accept the chronicity of pain. Acute medical model providers, like surgeons and interventional pain physicians, see their role as one in which they relieve pain. They tend to instill hope with such phrases as, "We'll get you patched up." Of course, they mean well. The implication, though, is clear: they believe a cure is forthcoming in the procedure that they'll deliver. As such, they fail to recognize the chronicity of the patient's pain and continue attempts to cure a pain disorder long after it could reasonably be considered chronic. As a result, they fail to refer patients to CPRPs.

A related possibility is that some providers still continue to conceptualize chronic pain as a symptom of long-lasting structural problems, such as in the spine, rather than a nervous system problem – central sensitization. As such, they refer patients to providers like surgeons and interventional pain physicians who attempt to treat structural problems in the spine, rather than CPRPs that treat central sensitization of the nervous system.

The healthcare system is currently in the process of changing our understanding of what chronic pain is. The conceptualization of it as a symptom of a long-lasting injury still holds sway. It's only been in the last few years that it has become increasingly clear that chronic pain is a disorder unto itself – a disorder of the nervous system attributable to central sensitization. It's not an exaggeration to say that something of a paradigm shift is occurring in the field of chronic pain management. Many healthcare providers haven't yet fully made the transition in their understanding and so continue to make recommendations for surgery and procedures that aim to modify the original injury or illness that started the pain – even if it's been years since the initial onset of pain.

Through no fault of their own, many patients are also unaware of this shift in understanding the nature of chronic pain. Understandably, the average person with chronic pain isn't an expert on the latest scientific advances in the field. As a consequence, they don't demand care that's most appropriate for the nervous system condition that they have – central sensitization. They simply get whatever care their providers recommend, trusting in the expertise of their providers. It's the luck of the draw as to whether they get referred to a provider who understands chronic pain as a disorder of the nervous system or as a symptom of a long-lasting injury or illness. If it's the latter type of provider, they typically won't get recommended to a CPRP.

Many commentators also cite financial reasons (cf. Schofferman, 2006; Taylor, 2011; Weiner & Levi, 2004). In the U. S., healthcare is a business. Individual providers are typically reimbursed per procedure or therapy they provide. It can't go unnoticed that the profit generated from surgeries and interventional procedures is dramatically larger and disproportionate to the amount of profit CPRPs can generate. So, to the question of why a referral to a CPRP didn't come earlier, would it be too cynical to answer with the old adage, 'Follow the money'? I'll leave it to the reader to decide.

As is evident, there may be a number of answers to the question as to why a referral never came earlier in the trajectory of a chronic pain patient's care. Almost inevitably, as patients near completion of their CPRP, and as they're getting better, we have this discussion of why and how they never got referred to the program earlier. I've come to see that it's an important step in the process. It's part of their adjustment to the new-found improvements in their well-being. They can't help but think that maybe they could have gotten better sooner, that they wouldn't have had to suffer for so long. They have to come to terms with what could have been.

It's important to spend some time on the issue of what-could-have-been, but not too much time. Yes, the system has its flaws and, yes, maybe at one point in the past you wouldn't have been ready to participate in a CPRP had it been recommended to you. It does no good, though, to get angry with yourself or with the flaws in the system. Rehabilitation is a process of becoming ready for change, making the changes, becoming good at them, and maintaining them. There is no universal timeline for achieving these stages in the process. So, don't spend too much time looking back at the past.

What's most important is your present state of well-being and maintaining it into the future. Accept ownership of the changes that you've made. You did it. Reflect upon it and feel the power that comes with taking back control.

Apprehensions that come with having a brighter future

With the progress they've made, patients who complete a CPRP commonly have to come to terms with one other thing. True, progress empowers them. They feel like they're finally back on track and they are going somewhere with their lives. And yet, they're also apprehensive. For all its benefits, change and progress is also a bit scary.

After all, by the time many patients participate in a CPRP, they've become somewhat adjusted to what they perceived would be their future – a long wait until a cure can be found. In Chapter Two, we called it a "holding pattern." Remember our friends Tom and Sarah? They were each in a holding pattern of being managed on long-term opioid medications and receiving disability. They were each waiting in this holding pattern until a cure could be found. Tom got used to the holding pattern, whereas Sarah didn't and so decided to get into a CPRP. Just like you, she got better and now has a future that doesn't require opioid medications or disability. This future typically takes some getting used to.

Successful completers of a CPRP now face a future that they didn't think they'd have. Even if it's disturbing and depressing, the status quo of the holding pattern was safe and familiar. You know what to expect. Now, though, you're getting better and are leaving the holding pattern. Maybe, you've begun volunteering somewhere, or returned to work part-time or you've already returned to full-time employment. You're also no longer taking opioid medications. You're excited and thrilled by your progress. Nonetheless, you can't help but have doubts: "Can I keep it going? What if…"

It's normal to have such apprehensions. A lot has changed and with such changes come risk. It's easy to start catastrophizing. Before you know it, you find yourself trying to get rid of pain by avoiding activities and believing that you can't work or do other activities outside the home or that you can't do any of these things without relying on opioid medications. Catastrophizing, fear-avoidance, and I-can't-thinking are so familiar. Such familiarity gives them the illusion of security. It seems safe to stay the same. Change can seem too full of risk.

Change is also full of possibilities – possibilities that you didn't think you could have. You've demonstrated it to yourself that you can achieve them. Recall that we started this book by imagining what it would be like to get back into the normal range of functioning despite having chronic pain. We imagined you being involved and engaged in your life, your work, and your relationships. We set out to become reasonably happy, not blissful, but as happy as anyone else is, even those without chronic pain. You're now well on your way. You've completed a CPRP and despite having chronic pain, you're feeling better, both physically and emotionally, and have become re-engaged in your life and your life's activities. Don't trade it all in for fear.

So, acknowledge that it's normal to be afraid. Observe your fears, and challenge them, just as you have been practicing in your program. Catch yourself catastrophizing and catch yourself in I-can't-thinking. Recognize that these beliefs just aren't true. Recognize that you're changing. You are already starting to live a normal life with chronic pain. The fact that you're already doing it demonstrates that you can. Unless some altogether different and unforeseen tragedy happens, tomorrow is going to be a lot like today. You have chronic pain. It doesn't change in radical, unforeseen ways overnight. Remind yourself of that and that you're succeeding in self-managing it. Tomorrow is going to be a lot like today and you're managing it well today.

Maintaining changes and finding balance

Let's review how you're going to maintain your gains. Follow these three broad guidelines:

1. attend any aftercare that your program provides;
2. develop a routine of self-management and stick to it;
3. practice maintaining balance in your life's pursuits.

CPRPs customarily have an aftercare component. Aftercare services are therapies that occur for patients following the completion of a CPRP. Aftercare typically consists of ongoing medication management (particularly when patients continue to taper opioids), access to exercise facilities for independent use, facilitated groups or classes for some specified period of time, and care coordination with patients' primary care providers.

Aftercare is important because it provides a bridge between the intensive, daily therapies of your CPRP and the independent self-management of the rest of your life. By the end of your program and for some time thereafter, you can see yourself as in a practicing phase of your self-management. You've likely learned much of what you'll learn, but you're still new at it. You're practicing the skills, getting the hang of them, and in the early stages of seeing results. It helps to be able to return to your CPRP providers for periodic coaching advice. Groups and classes where you meet up with other graduates of the program are also helpful in this regard. The group leaders reinforce what you've learned. You get to compare the successes and failures of your fellow graduates. In all, aftercare helps to maintain momentum of your progress and it's imperative that you take advantage of whatever aftercare your program offers.

It's also necessary to develop a routine for your self-management and make it part of your permanent lifestyle. In your program, you engaged in various ways to self-manage pain all day, every day, for three or four weeks. You won't be able to keep that schedule once you have completed the program. However, you need to remain engaged in some types of self-management on a regular basis.

With regard to the first prong of self-management, a good rule of thumb is that you should pick either a relaxation exercise or a mild aerobic exercise, such as walking, and do it on a daily basis; the relaxation exercise should be at least 20 minutes long and the mild aerobic exercise should be at least 30 minutes long; and then you should do the other exercise, whichever one you didn't pick, on an every other day basis. In the few weeks following completion of the program, experiment with the times that you engage in these activities. Eventually, you'll find times that work for you. Once finding these times, stick to them and make them part of your daily and weekly routine. Of course, you have to be realistic about it in order to balance other priorities. You may have to get up an hour earlier to get your walk in every day or walk on your lunch break at work, or have dinner a little later because you walk after work. Maybe, you engage in your relaxation exercise during one of these times. However you do it, stick to it and make it part of the structure of each day.

Patients who are successful with establishing a routine often engage in some helpful practices to ensure that they don't put off these self-management activities. For instance, they keep a weekly calendar or planner and they write in the times and days that they engage in their aerobic and relaxation exercises. In other words, they treat these exercises like appointments that they schedule the rest of their day's activities around. Other patients find people with whom to do their aerobic exercises. They've become accustomed to exercising in a group while in the CPRP and so they have their spouse or neighbor exercise with them. Maybe they continue their exercises with fellow patients from their CPRP at a local fitness center. These practices force you to be accountable for maintaining the changes that you've made: if you find yourself inclined to put off exercising one day, you'll get a call from your exercise partner, asking, "Where are you?"

The other lifestyle changes are important too. Continue with your reduced caffeine use and pursuit of quitting smoking, if either is applicable. Remain committed to a hot bath most every night as part of your bedtime routine. You need to maintain your sleep hygiene. Don't engage in stressful or exciting activities right before bed. Ensure that you go to bed at more or less the same time and get up at more or less at the same time. Your behaviors in all these ways serve to regulate your nervous system. With time, they become the new normal and your nervous system finds an improved balance.

With regard to the second prong of self-management, you need to continue to practice maintaining an observational self, recognizing your old and ineffective ways of reacting to pain, and changing them for the better. With practice, these better ways of reacting become your new automatic reactions.

While there's no schedule to practice coping with pain, you'll want to practice it every time you think of it. At this point, you may have sticky notes placed strategically around your house to remind you. Perhaps, you're carrying around an object in your pocket, which reminds you every time you touch it. With time, you simply become more and more self-observant and intentional about how you react to pain.

All these strategies help to establish a routine that becomes the new normal. At first, it takes a lot of effort to maintain focus on these new lifestyle behaviors and coping skills. As you continue, however, they'll take less effort to do them. In fact, you'll continue to feel physically and emotionally better and your improved well-being comes to motivate you to continue. It becomes self-motivating.

There doesn't seem to be an established timeline in which it will happen. It might be a month or six months. You may not even know when it happens. It's like you cross a threshold that makes a big difference, but which comes with no fanfare and you don't even notice that you crossed it. You don't know it until something happens that prevents you from engaging in your aerobic exercise or relaxation exercise and you come to realize that you miss your exercise! You feel sore or stiff or maybe you feel a little more nervous or irritable or depressed. Initially, you don't know what happened, but then you make the connection: you haven't got to your exercises for a few days! You subsequently recognize how much you have come to rely on these healthy lifestyle changes. They are no longer new. They are part of how you now live.

The threshold that marks the new normal points to the fact that you've developed a better balance in your life. Maintaining this balance is the third thing that is imperative to do when successfully self-managing pain for the rest of your life.

You started to read this book and participate in a CPRP because you wanted a better life and you saw that getting better at managing chronic pain was the way to do it. After all, your chronic pain was leading to many problems in your life. It stood to reason that to improve these problems you had to get better at managing their cause, namely, your chronic pain. Now, you've completed a CPRP and are well on your way to managing pain better than you ever have in the past. As a result, life is picking up. You are back at work or some other meaningful activity. You are more socially active and you are engaging in recreational activities. You are even enjoying them more than you have in a long time. Your mood has improved and you are more confident. You feel like you are getting back into the swing of things. Your overall life has gotten better and a whole lot less stressful because you have gotten better at managing chronic pain.

Now, remember, though, you have a chronic pain syndrome. Chronic pain syndromes are pain disorders that are complicated by stressors. The chronic pain may have caused these stressors, but these stressors also further exacerbate the pain. So, while it's true that you can reduce life's stressors by getting better at managing chronic pain, it's also true that to continue to improve your pain management, you have to get better at managing life's stressors. Here's the way to think about it: your life gets better when you manage chronic pain well, but your chronic pain gets better when you manage life well.

Another way to look at it is to see the issue in terms of the nervous system. Chronic pain is largely the result of the nervous system being stuck in a persistent, or regulated, state of reactivity. The heightened sensitivities of the nervous system are now maintaining pain itself. The nervous system, though, is also responsible for regulating our emotional life. With the nervous system stuck in a heightened state of reactivity, patients are commonly emotionally reactive: they are anxious or frustrated easily or irritable or tearful easily or depressed. You've learned that to manage chronic pain well you have to down-regulate your nervous system. Once you do, you have less pain, but also less emotional problems.

Now, additionally, the nervous system also reflects, at least in part, what goes on around you. In Chapter Four, we learned that stressful events affect the nervous system, making it more reactive, via the stress response. Relationships and activities can either stress or calm the nervous system. So, in other words, to manage chronic pain well, you have to manage your nervous system and, to do the latter, you also have to manage the stressors of your life.

From this vantage point, we can see the importance of maintaining balance. When life gets out of whack, your nervous system gets out of whack and your pain flares. Regulating your life is thus a way to down-regulate your nervous system.

So, moderate your activities and pace them. Don't find yourself engaging in perfectionistic and workaholic behaviors. Manage workload. Good is good enough. Don't get too far out into any extreme and if you do, catch yourself, notice it, and reel yourself back in. Get back into your routines. In doing so, you maintain a healthy balance across all the domains of your life: physical, emotional, relational, work, and lifestyle. By keeping your life in moderation, you maintain your pain in moderation.

Pain levels are a barometer of how you're managing your life

From here, we can introduce one more advanced coping strategy before bringing this book to a close. Because you have chronic pain, you are apt to always have some level of pain. However, your pain level on any given day is largely determined by what else is going on in your life and how well you are coping with it (i.e., regulating it). Some days, your pain is minimal. On other days, it's your usual baseline level of pain. On still other days, you experience the high levels of a pain flare. As we've discussed, what largely determines your pain level at any given time is how reactive your nervous system is and how you're coping.

Patients commonly report that while on vacation their pain is quite manageable, even minimal. During the usual course of their lives, they commonly say that their pain is at their usual level, fluctuating one or two points on a 0-10 scale. At times like the hectic holidays or planning for an adult child's wedding or when a spouse loses a job and is now hanging around the house all day, patients commonly report high levels of pain. The lesson here is that chronic pain levels reflect, at least in part, how you're managing what's going on in life.

In other words, people who cope with pain well tend to see their chronic pain as a barometer. Pain levels convey something important about how you're managing the stressors of life. When you stay on top of the stressors and orchestrate your life to minimize them, pain levels tend to be minimized. When stressors get the best of you or when you lead a life that's too hectic, then pain levels tend to be maximized. Chronic pain levels are thus a barometer of how you're doing in managing your health and life.

The use of the barometer metaphor changes your relationship with pain. Prior to participating in a CPRP, your relationship to pain was apt to be something like the following: you were trying to get rid of it or avoid it, and it distressed you – you were anxious, angry, or depressed about it. In effect, the relationship was one of waging war on pain and you were tending to lose each battle. Since participating in a CPRP, however, you've been changing your relationship to chronic pain. You've been changing it to something like the following: managing it, controlling it, ignoring it, but also becoming acquainted with it, no longer becoming alarmed by it, and learning how to live with it. In other words, you've been learning how to make peace with it and live together. Now, with the use of the barometer metaphor, you can change your relationship a step further. Your chronic pain levels provide you with helpful feedback about how you're living life.

Maybe, now, you can become curious about your chronic pain. It's providing you with helpful information. Receive the information and use it in an open and light-hearted way. Don't get down on yourself if you have a pain flare. Rather, accept it and be curious about it. It's your barometer and you can use the information it provides to make decisions about how to lead a healthier, happier, and less painful life.

Concluding Remarks

You've come a long way. Yes, you've come a long way to be able to tolerate this discussion of the barometer metaphor. In Chapter Two, we defined coming to cope better as a change in your perspective on a problem. It doesn't so much change the problem you have, you still have it, but you see it in a new light. This change in perspective makes a big difference. It makes the problem less problematic. You can deal with it better. It's no longer impairing.

In the case of chronic pain, you've come to accept it and make peace with it. With the use of the barometer metaphor, you now use it to your benefit. Of course, you never would have chosen to have chronic pain, but now that you have it, you recognize that you can use it. You see that it gives you feedback on how you are doing in terms of your overall well-being. It gives you, at any given time, feedback on how well you are coping and how much stress you're experiencing. In other words, it gives you information on how well-regulated your life is – the degree to which you keep it in balance. It's important information to use in your day-to-day life as you self-manage chronic pain.

Had you not participated in a CPRP or read this book, it's unlikely that you would've been able to tolerate this discussion. That's the thing about coping and coming to cope better. It's a process. It's a process of developing what psychologists call *ego strength*. Ego strength is the capacity to maintain an observational self while at the same time tolerating feedback about yourself without a high degree of sensitivity. Throughout your chronic pain rehabilitation, you've been developing ego strength. You've been slowly accepting more and more feedback about your pain and yourself, observing it in yourself, reflecting on it, learning from it, and making changes on account of it. The fact that you can tolerate this discussion of the barometer metaphor, reflect on it, learn from it, and apply it, indicates that you've come a long way.

It's easy to imagine that those who have yet to go through this process would become upset by the discussion of the barometer metaphor. They could easily take it as invalidating the legitimacy of their pain because they see their pain as solely a medical problem over which they have no control and therefore no responsibility in its management. They could also hear the metaphor as blaming them for their pain. As such, it's easy to imagine that they'd become angry with it, reject it, and reject us, if we were to bring it up with them. It's not that they're mistaken. It's not that we're mistaken. It's that our timing is off. The use of the barometer metaphor implies a way of making sense of chronic pain for which they are simply not yet ready.

It would be like if we helped students with a complicated, multi-step math problem by telling them about the last few steps in the problem, when what they really needed was a review of the first few steps to simply get them started. We're not actually wrong in telling them about the last few steps, but we're not being very helpful either. They need help with the beginning steps, not the ending steps, of the problem.

The fact that you can tolerate and learn from the use of the barometer metaphor points to something important about you. You are no longer in the beginning stages of taking back control of your life. When experiencing a pain flare, you can see that it tells you that you have gotten off your routines and your life has become a little too hectic, or dysregulated. You can subsequently use the information to make changes in how you're coping and managing the stressors of life. All of it is to imply that you can tolerate the recognition that you in fact have some modest degree of control over your pain when you practice the skills of self-management over time. This recognition isn't seen as invalidating or blaming. It's rather empowering. Despite having chronic pain, you have learned to self-manage it well. You have re-engaged in the activities of life: work, family, social and recreational activities. You have become reasonably happy, at least as happy as most anyone else is. In other words, you now have hope even when there is no cure.

References

Alexander, J., DeVries, A., Kigerl, K., Dahlman, J., & Popovich, P. (2009). Stress exacerbates neuropathic pain via glucocorticoid and NMDA receptor activation.
Brain, Behavior and Immunity, 23, 851-860.

Allen, D. B., & Waddell, G. (1989). An historical perspective on low back pain and disability. *Acta Orthopaedica Scandinavica 60, (Suppl. 234)*, 1-23.

American Academy of Pain Medicine and the American Pain Society. (1997). The use of opioids for the treatment of chronic pain: . *The Clinical Journal of Pain, 13*, 6-8.

American Psychiatric Association. (1994). *Diagnostic and statistical manual of mental disorders* (4th ed.). Washington DC: Author.

Andersson, G. B. (1999). Epidemiological features of chronic low-back pain. *The Lancet, 354*, 581-585.

Angst, M. & Clark, J. (2006). Opioid-induced hyperalgesia: A quantitative systematic review. *Anesthesiology, 104*, 570-587.

Antonuccio, D. O., & Danton, W. G. (1995). Psychotherapy versus medication for depression: Challenging conventional wisdom with data. *Professional Psychology: Research & Practice, 26*, 574-586.

Arden, N. K., Price, C., Reading, I., Stubbing, J., Hazelgrove, J., Dunne, C... Cooper C. (2005). A multicentre randomized controlled trial of epidural corticosteroid injections for sciatica: The WEST study. *Rheumatology, 44*, 1399-1406.

Arendt-Nielsen, L., Nie, H., Laursen M. B., Laursen, B. S., Madeleine P., Simonson O. H., & Graven-Nielsen, T. (2010). Sensitization in patients with painful knee osteoarthritis. *Pain, 149*, 573-581.

Arneberg, P., Bjertness, E., Storhaug. K., Glennas, A., & Bjerkhoel, F. (1992). Remaining teeth, oral dryness and dental health habits in rheumatoid arthritis patients. *Community Dental and Oral Epidemiology, 20,* 292-295.

Arroll, B., Macgillivrary, S., Ogston, S., Reid, I., Sullivan, F., Williams, B., & Crombie, I. (2005). Efficacy and tolerability of tricyclic antidepressants and SSRI's compared with placebo for treatment of depression in primary care: A meta-analysis. *Annals of Family Medicine, 3,* 449-456.

Bajaj, P., Bajaj, P., Madsen, H., & Arendt-Nielsen, L. (2003). Endometriosis is associated with central sensitization: A psycho-physical controlled study. *The Journal of Pain, 4,* 372-380.

Baliki, M. N., Chialvo, D. R., Geha, P. Y., Levy, R. M., Harden, R. N., Parrish, T. B., & Apkarian, A. V. (2006). Chronic pain and the emotional brain: Specific brain activity associated with spon-taneous fluctuations of intensity of chronic back pain. *Journal of Neuroscience, 26,* 12165-12173.

Banic, B, Petersen-Felix, S., Andersen O. K., Radanov, B. P., Villiger, P. M., Arendt-Nielsen, L., & Curatolo, M. (2004). Evidence for spinal cord hypersensitivity in chronic pain after whiplash injury and fibromyalgia. *Pain, 107,* 7-15.

Bendix, A. F., Bendix, T., Lund, C., Kirkbak, S., & Ostenfeld, S. (1997). Comparisons of three intensive programs for chronic low back pain patients: A prospective, randomized, observer-blinded study with one year follow-up. *Scandinavian Journal of Rehabilitation Medicine, 29,* 81-89.

Bendtsen, L. (2000). Central sensitization in tension-type headaches – possible pathophysiological mechanisms. *Cephalalgia, 20,* 486-508.

Benarroch, E. E. (2006). Pain-autonomic interactions. *Neurological Sciences, 27,* s130-s133.

Bhatia, V, & Tandon, R. K. (2005). Stress and the gastrointestinal tract. *Journal of Gastroenterology and Hepatology, 20,* 332-339.

Blackburn-Munro, G. (2008). Hypothalamo-pituitary-adrenal axis dysfunction as a contributory factor to chronic pain and depres-sion. *Current Pain and Headache Reports, 8,* 116-124.

Blumner, K. H., & Marcus, S. C. (2009). Changing perceptions of depression: Ten-year trends from the general social survey. *Psychiatric Services, 60*, 306-312.

Boos, N., Semmer, N., Elfering, A., Schade, V. Gal, I., Kissling, R... Main, C. J. (2000). Natural history of individuals with asymptomatic abnormalities on magnetic resonance imaging: Predictors of low back pain-related medical consultation and work incapacity. *Spine, 25*, 1484-1492.

Breivek, H., Collett, B., Ventfridda, V., Cohen, R., & Gallacher, D. (2006). Survey of chronic pain in Europe: Prevalence, impact on daily life, and treatment. *European Journal of Pain, 10*, 287-333.

Buscemi, N., Vandermeer, B., Friesen, C., Bialy, L., Tubman, M., Ospina, M...Witmans, M. (2007). The efficacy and safety of drug treatments for chronic insomnia in adults: A meta-analysis of RCTs. *Journal of General Internal Medicine, 22*, 1335-1350.

Carragee, E., Alamin, T., Cheng, I., Franklin, T., & Hurwitz, E. (2006). Does minor trauma cause serious low back illness? *Spine, 31*, 2942-2949.

Carragee, E. J., Alamin, T. F., Miller, J. L., & Carragee, J. M. (2005). Discographic, MRI and psychosocial determinants of low back pain disability and remission: A prospective study in subjects with benign persistent back pain. *Spine, 5*, 24-35.

Cassidy, J. D., Carroll, L., & Cote, P. (1998). The Saskatchewan health and back pain survey: The prevalence of low back pain and related disability in Saskatchewan adults. *Spine, 23*, 1860-1866.

Chabel, C., Erjavec, M., Jacobson, L., Mariano, A., & Chaney, E. (1997). Prescription opiate abuse in chronic pain patients: Clinical criteria, incidence and predictors. *Clinical Journal of Pain, 13*, 150-155.

Chapman, C. R., Tuckett, R. P., & Song, C. W. (2008). Pain and stress in a systems perspective: Reciprocal neural, endocrine and immune interactions. *Journal of Pain, 9*, 122-145.

Chen, L., Malarick, C., Seefeld, L., Wang, S., Houghton, & Mao, J. (2009). Altered quantitative sensory testing outcome in subjects with opioid therapy. *Pain, 143*, 65-70.

Chen, W., Wang, S., Fuh, J., Lin, C., Ko, Y., & Lin Y. (2011). Persistent ictal-like visual cortical excitability in chronic migraine. *Pain, 152*, 254-258.

Chiang, Y., Hung, T., Lee, C., Yan, J., & Ho, I. (2010). Enhancement of tolerance development to morphine in rats prenatally exposed to morphine, methadone, and buprenorphine. *Journal of Biomedical Science, 17*, 46.

Chouinard, G. (2004). Issues in the clinical use of benzodiazepines: Potency, withdrawal, and rebound. *Journal of Clinical Psychiatry, 65*, Suppl 5, 7-12.

Chua, n. H., Van Suijlekom, H. A., Vissers, K. C., Arendt-Nielsen, L., & Wilder-Smith, O. H. (2011). Differences in sensory processing between chronic cervical zygapophysial joint pain patients with and without cervicogenic headache. *Cephalalgia, 31*, 953-963.

Cohen, S., & Lichtenstein, E. (1990). Perceived stress, quitting smoking, and smoking relapse. *Health Psychology, 9*, 466-478.

Cortelli, P, & Pierangeli, G. (2003). Chronic pain-autonomic interactions. *Neurological Sciences, 24*, s68-s70.

Cote, P., Cassidy, J. D., & Carroll, L. (1998). The Saskatchewan health and back pain survey: The prevalence of neck pain and related disability in Saskatchewan adults. *Spine, 23*, 1689-1698.

Crombez, G., Vlaeyen, J. W., Heuts, P. H., & Lysens, R. (1999). Pain-related fear is more disabling than pain itself: Evidence on the role of pain-related fear in chronic back pain disability. *Pain, 80*, 329-339.

Curatolo, M., Arendt-Nielsen, L., & Petersen-Felix, S. (2006). Central hypersensitivity in chronic pain: Mechanisms and clinical implications. *Physical Medicine and Rehabilitation Clinics of North America, 17*, 287-302.

Denison, E., Asenlof, P., & Lindberg, P. (2004). Self-efficacy, fear avoidance, and pain intensity as predictors of disability in subacute and chronic musculoskeletal pain patients in primary health care. *Pain, 111*, 245-252.

DeRubeis, R. J., Gelfand, L. A., Tang, T. Z., & Simons, A. D. (1999). Medications versus cognitive behavior therapy for severely depressed outpatients: Meta-analysis of four randomized comparisons. *American Journal of Psychiatry, 156*, 1007-1013.

Dobson, K. S., Hollon, S. D., Dimidjian, S., Schmaling, K. B., Kohlenberg, R. J., Gallop, R... Jacobson, N. S. (2008). Randomized trial of behavioral activation, cognitive therapy, and antidepressant medication in the prevention of relapse and recurrence in major depression. *Journal of Clinical and Consulting Psychology, 76*, 468-477.

Duric, V., & McCarson, K. E. (2006). Persistent pain produces stress-like alterations in hipocampal neurogenesis and gene expression. *Journal of Pain, 7*, 544-555.

Endean, A., Palmer, K. T., & Coggon, D. (2011). Potential of MRI findings to refine case definition for mechanical low back pain in epidemiological studies: A systematic review. *Spine, 36*, 160-169.

Fanciulo, G. J., Ball, P. A., Girault, G., Rose, R. J., Hanson, B., & Weinstein, J. N. (2002). An observational study on the prevalence and pattern of opioid use in 25, 479 patients with spine and radicular pain. *Spine, 27*, 201-205.

Fernandez-Lao, C., Cantarero-Villanueva, I., Fernandez-de-Las-Penas, C, Del-Moral-Avila, R., Arendt-Nielsen, L., Arroyo-Morales, M. (2010). Myofascial trigger points in neck and shoulder muscles and widespread pressure pain hypersensitivity in patients with post-mastectomy pain: Evidence of peripheral and central sensitization. *Clinical Journal of Pain, 26*, 798-806.

Finan, P. H., Buenaver, L. F., Bounds, S. C., Hussain, S., Park, R. J., Haque, U. J...Smith, M. T. (2013). Discordance between pain and radiographic severity in knee osteoarthritis: Findings from quantitative sensory testing of central sensitization. *Arthritis & Rheumatism, 65(2)*, 363-372. doi: 10.1002/art.34646

Fournier, J. C., DeRubeis, R. J., Hollon, S. D., Dimidjian, S., Amsterdam, J. D., Shelton, R. C., & Fawcett, J. (2010). Antidepressant drug effects and depression severity. *Journal of the American Medical Association, 303,* 47-53.

Gatchel, R., J., & Okifuji, A. (2006). Evidence-based scientific data documenting the treatment and cost-effectiveness of comprehensive pain programs for chronic non-malignant pain. *Journal of Pain, 7,* 779-793.

Gatchel, R. J., Polatin, P. B., & Mayer, T. G. (1995). The dominant role of psychosocial risk factors in the development of chronic low back pain disability. *Spine, 20,* 2072-2079.

Gibson J. N., & Waddell, G. (Updated January 6, 2007). Surgical intervention for lumbar disc prolapse. [Cochrane Review]. In *Cochrane Database of Systematic Reviews,* 2007 (2). Retrieved November 25, 2011, from The Cochrane Library, Wiley Interscience.

Giesecke, T, Gracely, R. H., Grant, M. A., Nachemson, A., Petzke, F., Williams, D. A., & Clauw, D. J. (2004). Evidence of augmented central pain processing in idiopathic chronic low back pain. *Arthritis and Rheumatism, 50,* 613-623.

Gould, R. A., Otto, M. W., Pollack, M. H., & Yap, L. (1997). Cognitive behavioral and pharmacological treatment of generalized anxiety disorder: A preliminary meta-analysis. *Behavior Therapy, 28,* 285-305.

Graham, C. H., & Meechan, J. G. (2005). Dental management of patients taking methadone. *Dental Update, 32,* 481-482.

Gureje, O, Simon, G. E., & Von Korff, M. (2001). A cross-national study of the course of persistent pain in primary care. *Pain, 92,* 195-200.

Hall, A. M., Kamper, S. J., Maher, C. G., Latimer, J., Ferreira, M. L., & Nicholas, M. K. (2011). Symptoms of depression and stress mediate the effect of pain on disability. *Pain, 152,* 1044-1051.

Hauser, W., Bernardy, K., Uceyler, N., & Sommer, C. (2009). Treatment of fibromyalgia syndrome with antidepressants: A meta-analysis. *Journal of the American Medical Association, 301,* 198-209.

Hay, J., White, J., Booner, F., Somogyi, A., Semple, T., & Rounsefell, B. (2009). Hyperalgesia in opioid-managed chronic pain and opioid-dependent patients. *Journal of Pain, 10,* 316-322.

Henschke, N., Ostelo, R. W., van Tulder, M. W., Valaeyen, J. W., Linton, S. J., Morley, S. J... Main, C. J. Behavioral treatment for chronic low back pain. [Cochrane Review]. In *Cochrane Database of Systematic Reviews*, 2010 (7). Retrieved November 26, 2011, from The Cochrane Library, Wiley Interscience.

Herbette, G. & Rime, B. (2004). Verbalization of emotion in chronic pain patients and their psychological adjustment. *Journal of Health Psychology, 9*, 661-676.

Heuzenroeder, L., Donnelly, M., Haby, M. M., Mihalopoulos, C., Rossell, R., Carter, R... Vos, T. (2004). Cost-effectiveness of psychological and pharmacological interventions for generalized anxiety disorder and panic disorder. *Australian and New Zealand Journal of Psychiatry, 38*, 602-612.

Hollon, S. D., Stewart, M. O., & Strunk, D. (2006). Enduring effects of cognitive behavioral therapy in the treatment of depression and anxiety. *Annual Review of Psychology, 57*, 285-315.

Hollon, S. D., DeRubeis, R. J., Shleton R. C., Amsteram, J. D., Saloman, R. M., O'Reardon, J. D... Gallop. R. (2005). Prevention of relapse following cognitive therapy versus medications in moderate to severe depression. *Archives of General Psychiatry, 62*, 417-422.

Hughes, J. R. (1992). Tobacco withdrawal in self quitters. *Journal of Consulting and Clinical Psychology, 60*, 689-697.

Humphreys, S. C., Hodges, S. D., Patwardhan, A., Eck, J. C., Covington, L. A., & Sartori, M. (1998). The natural history of the cervical foramen in symptomatic and asymptomatic individuals aged 20-60 years as measured by magnetic resonance imaging: A descriptive approach. *Spine, 23*, 2180-2184.

Hutton, M. J., Baker, J. H., & Powell, J. M. (2011). Modic vertebral body changes: The natural history as assessed by consecutive magnetic resonance imaging. *Spine, 36*, 2304-2307.

Jarvik, J. G., Hollingworth, W., Heagerty, P. J., Haynor, D. R., Boyko, E. J., & Deyo, R. A. (2005) Three-year incidence of low back pain in an initially asymptomatic cohort. *Spine, 30*, 1541-1548.

Jensen, M. C., Brant-Zawadzki, M. N., Obuchowski, N., Modic, M. T., Malkasian, D., Ross, J. S. (1994). Magnetic resonance imaging of the lumbar spine in people without back pain. *New England Journal of Medicine, 331*, 69-73.

Ji, G., Fu, Y., Ruppert, K. A., & Neugebauer, V. (2007). Pain-related anxiety-like behavior requires CRF1 receptors in the amygdala. *Molecular Pain, 3*, 13.

Kales, A., Soldatos, C. R., Bixler, E. O., & Kales, K. O. (1983). Rebound insomnia and rebound anxiety: A review. *Pharmacology, 26*, 121-137.

Kamboj, Tookman, A., Jones, L. & Curran, H. V. (2005). The effect of immediate-release morphine on cognitive functioning in patients receiving chronic opioid therapy in palliative care. *Pain, 117*, 388-395.

Karjalainen, K, A., Malmivaara, A., van Tulder, M. W., Roine, R., Jauhiainen, M., Hurri, H., Koes, B. W. Multidisciplinary bio-psychosocial rehabilitation for subacute low back pain among working age adults. [Cochrane Review]. In *Cochrane Database of Systematic Reviews*, 2003 (2). Retrieved November 26, 2011, from The Cochrane Library, Wiley Interscience.

Katz, N. & Mazer, N. A., (2009). The impact of opioids on the endocrine system. *Clinical Journal of Pain, 25*, 170-175.

Kirsch, I., Deacon, B. J., Huedo-Medina, T. B., Scoboria, A., Moore, T. J., & Johnson, B. T. (2008). Initial severity and antidepressant benefits: A meta-analysis of data submitted to the Food and Drug Administration. *PLoS Medicine, 5*, e45.

Klauenberg, S., Maier, C., Assion, H., Hoffmann, A., Krumova, E. K., Magerl, W., Scherens, A., Treede, R. & Juckel. (2008). Depression and changed pain perception: Hints for a central disinhibition mechanism. *Pain, 140*, 332-343.

Knoeller, S. M., Seifried, C. (2000). Historical perspective: History of spinal surgery. *Spine, 25*, 2838-2843.

Kodama, D., Ono, H., & Tanabe, M. (2011). Increased hippocampal glycine uptake and cognitive dysfunction after peripheral nerve injury. *Pain, 152,* 809-817.

Kuehl, L. K., Michaux, G. P., Richter, S., Schachinger, H., & Anton F. (2010). Increased basal mechanical sensitivity but decreased perceptual wind-up in a human model of relative hypocortisolism. *Pain, 194,* 539-546.

Lacasse, J. R. (2005). Consumer advertising of psychiatric medications biases the public against nonpharmacological treatment. *Ethical and Human Psychology and Psychiatry, 7,* 175-179.

Latremoliere, A., & Woolf, C. J. (2009). Central sensitization: A generator of pain hypersensitivity by central neural plasticity. *Journal of Pain, 10,* 895-926.

Lim, G., Wang, S., Zeng, Q., Sung, B., & Mao, J. (2005). Evidence for a long-term influence on morphine tolerance after previous exposure: Role of neuronal glucoticoid receptors. *Pain, 114,* 81-92.

Linton, S. J., & Buer, N. (1995). Working despite pain: Factors associated with work attendance versus dysfunction. *International Journal of Behavior Medicine, 2,* 252-262.

Lorduy, K. M., Liegey-Dougall, A., Haggard, R., Sanders, C. N., & Gatchel, R. J. (2013). The prevalence of comorbid symptoms of central sensitization syndrome among three different groups of temporomandibular disorder patients. *Pain Practice.* Advance online publication. doi: 10.1111/papr.12029.

Mahlla, A., Ciampi de Andrade, D., Baudic, S., Perrot, S., & Bouhassira, D. (2010). Alteration in cortical excitability in patients with fibromyalgia. *Pain, 149,* 495-500.

Mao, J., Sung, B., Ji, R., & Lim, G. (2002). Neuronal apoptosis associated with morphine tolerance: Evidence for an opioid-induced neurotoxic mechanism. *Journal of Neuroscience, 22,* 7650-7661.

Martell, B. A., O'Connor, P. G., Kerns, R. D., Becker, W. C., Morales, K. H., Kosten, T. R., Fiellin. D. A. (2007). Systematic review: Opioid treatment for chronic back pain: Prevalence, efficacy, and association with addiction. *Annals of Internal Medicine, 146,* 116-127.

Mathew, S. J., & Charney, D. S. (2009). Publication bias and the efficacy of antidepressants. *American Journal of Psychiatry, 166,* 140-145.

Matsubara, Y., Kato, F., Mimatsu, K., Kajino, G., Nakamura, S., & Nitta, H. (1995). Serial changes on MRI in lumbar disc herniations treated conservatively. *Neuroradiology, 37,* 378-383.

Mayer, E. A. (2000). The neurobiology of stress and gastrointestinal disease. *Gut, 47,* 861-869.

Mayer, E. A., Naliboff, B. D., Chang, L., & Coutinho, S. V. (2001). V. Stress and irritable bowel syndrome. *American Journal of Physiology: Gastrointestinal and Liver Physiology, 280,* G519-G524.

McDonnell, D. E. (2004). History of spinal surgery: One neurosurgeon's perspective. *Neurosurgical Focus, 16,* 1-5.

McEwan, B. S. (2004). Protection and damage from acute and chronic stress: Allostasis and allostatic load and relevance to the pathophysiology of psychiatric disorders. *Annals of the New York Academy of Sciences, 1032,* 1-7.

McLean, S., Clauw, D., J., Abelson, J. L., & Liberzon, I. (2005). The development of persistent pain and psychological morbidity after motor vehicle collision: Integrating the potential role of stress response systems into a biopsychosocial model. *Psychosomatic Medicine, 67,* 783-790.

Meeus M., & Nijs, J. (2007). Central sensitization: A biopsychosocial explanation for chronic widespread pain in patients with fibromyalgia and chronic fatigue syndrome. *Clinical Journal of Rheumatology, 26,* 465-473.

Meeus M., Vervisch, S., De Clerck, L. S., Moorkens, G., Hans, G., & Nijs, J. (2012). Central sensitization in patients with rheumatoid arthritis: A systematic literature review. *Seminars in Arthritis & Rheumatism, 41,* 556-567.

Melzack, R., Coderre, T. J., Kat, J., & Vaccarino, A. L. (2001). Central neuroplasticity and pathological pain. *Annals of the New York Academy of Sciences, 933*, 157-174.

Mintzer. M. Z., & Stitzer, M. L. (2002). Cognitive impairment in methadone maintenance patients. *Drug and Alcohol Dependence, 67*, 41-51.

Mitra, S. (2008). Opioid-induced hyperalgesia: Pathophysiology and clinical implications. *Journal of Opioid Management, 4*, 123-130.

Mitte, K. (2005). A meta-analysis of the efficacy of psycho- and pharmacotherapy in panic disorder with and without agoraphobia. *Journal of Affective Disorders, 88*, 27-45.

Moncrieff, J, & Kirsch, I. (2005). Efficacy of antidepressants in adults. *British Medical Journal, 331*, 155-157.

Neugebauer, V., Li, W., Bird, G. C., & Han, J. S. (2004). The amygdala and persistent pain. *Neuroscientist, 10*, 221-234.

Ng, L., Chaudhary, N., & Sell, P. (2005). The efficacy of corticosteroids in periradicular infiltration in chronic radicular pain: A randomized, double-blind, controlled trial. *Spine, 30*, 857-862.

Nutt, D. J. (2005). Overview of diagnosis and drug treatments of anxiety disorders. *CNS Spectrum, 10*, 49-56.

O'Neill, S., Manniche, C., Graven-Nielsen, T., Arendt-Nielsen, L. (2007). Generalized deep-tissue hyperalgesia in patients with chronic low-back pain. *European Journal of Pain, 11*, 415-420.

Otto, M. W., Smits, J. A., & Reese, H. E. (2005). Combined psychotherapy for mood and anxiety disorders in adults: A review and analysis. *Clinical Psychology: Science and Practice, 12*, 72-86.

Pega, J. M., Sousa, J. C., Almeida, O. F., & Sousa, N. (2010). Stress and the neuroendocrinology of anxiety disorders. *Current Topics in Behavioral Neurosciences, 2*, 97-117.

Pennebaker J. W. (1997). *Opening up: The healing power of expressing emotion.* (New York: Guilford Press.)

Pennebaker J. W. & Chung, C. K. (2011). Expressive writing and its links to mental and physical health. In H. S. Friedman

(Ed.), *Oxford handbook of health psychology*. New York, NY: Oxford University Press.

Phillips, K. & Clauw, D. J. (2011). Central pain mechanisms in chronic pain states –maybe it is all in their head. *Best Practice Research in Clinical Rheumatology, 25*, 141-154.

Powell, M. C., Szypryt, P., Wilson, M., Symonds, E. M., & Worthington, B. S. (1986). Prevalence of lumbar disc degeneration observed by magnetic resonance in symptomless women. *The Lancet, 328*, 1366-1367.

Power, K. G., Jerrom, D. W., Simpson R. J., & Mitchell, M. (1985). Controlled study of withdrawal and rebound anxiety after six weeks of diazepam for generalized anxiety disorder. *British Medical Journal, 290*, 1246-1248

Prosser, J., Cohen, L. J., Steinfeld, M., Eisenberg, D., London, E. D., & Galynker, I. I. (2006). Neuropsychological functioning in opiate-dependent subjects receiving and following methadone maintenance treatment. *Drug and Alcohol Dependence, 84*, 240-247.

Ram, K. C., Eisenberg, E., Haddad, M., & Pud, D. (2008). Oral opioid use alters DNIC but not cold pain perception in patients with chronic pain – New perspective of opioid-induced hyperalgesia. *Pain, 139*, 431-438.

Reece, A. S. (2007). Dentition of addiction in Queensland: Poor dental status and major contributing drugs. *Australian Dental Journal, 52*, 144-149.

Rynn, M. A., Brawman-Mintzer, O. (2004). Generalized anxiety disorder: Acute and chronic treatment. *CNS Spectrums, 9*, 716-723.

Saarto T. & Wiffen, P. J. (Updated August 15, 2007). Antidepressants for neuropathic pain. [Cochrane Review]. In *Cochrane Database of Systematic Reviews*, 2007 (4). Retrieved November 12, 2011, from The Cochrane Library, Wiley Interscience.

Salerno, S. M., Browning, R., & Jackson, J. L. (2002). The effect of antidepressant treatment in chronic low-back pain: A meta-analysis. *Archives of Internal Medicine, 162*, 19-24.

Savage, R. A., Whitehouse, G. H., & Roberts, N. (1997). The relationship between magnetic resonance imaging appearance of the lumbar spine and low back pain, age, and occupation in males. *European Spine Journal, 6,* 106-114.

Schofferman, J. (2006). Interventional pain medicine: Financial success and ethical practice: An oxymoron? *Pain Medicine, 7, 5,* 457-460.

Shedler, J. (2010). The efficacy of psychodynamic psychotherapy. *American Psychologist, 65,* 98-109.

Social Security Online. (2011). Disability programs. Retrieved from http://www.ssa.gov/disability/professionals/blue-book/1.00-Musculoskeletal-Adult.htm#1_02.

Spielman, G. I., Berman, M. I., Usitalo, A. N. (2011). Psychotherapy versus second-generation antidepressants in the treatment of depression: A meta-analysis. *Journal of Nervous and Mental Disease, 199,* 142-149.

Stankewitz, A., & May, A. (2009). The phenomenon of changes in cortical excitability in migraine is not migraine-specific – A unifying thesis. *Pain, 145,* 14-17.

Staud, R. (2006). Biology and therapy of fibromyalgia: Pain in fibromyalgia syndrome. *Arthritis Research and Therapy, 8,* 208.

Sullivan, M. J., Lynch, M. E., & Clark, A. J. (2005). Dimensions of catastrophic thinking associated with pain experience and disability in patients with neuropathic pain conditions. *Pain, 113,* 310-315.

Sullivan, M. J., Stanish, W., Waite, H., Sullivan, M. & Tripp, D. A. (1998). Catastrophizing, pain, and disability in patients with soft-tissue injuries. *Pain, 77,* 253-260.

Symmons, D. P., van Hemert, A. M., Vandenbroucke, J. P., & Valkenburg, H. A. (1991). A longitudinal study of back pain and radiological changes in the lumbar spines of middle aged women. II. Radiographic findings. *Annals of the Rheumatic Diseases, 50,* 162-166.

Takatalo, J., Karppinen, J., Niinimaki, J., Taimela, S., Nayha, S., Jarvelin, M. R... Tervonen, O. (2009). Prevalence of degenerative imaging findings in lumbar magnetic imaging among young adults. *Spine, 34,* 1716-1721.

Taylor, M. L. (2011). The impact of the "business" of pain medicine on patient care. *Pain Medicine, 12, 5,* 763-772.

Toblin, R. L., Mack, K. A., Perveen, G., & Paulozzi, L. J. (2011). A population-based survey of chronic pain and its treatment with prescription drugs. *Pain, 152,* 1249-1255.

Turk, D. C. (2002). Clinical effectiveness and cost-effectiveness of treatments for patients with chronic pain. *The Clinical Journal of Pain, 18,* 355-365.

Turner, J. A., Jensen, M. P., & Romano, J. M. (2000). Do beliefs, coping, and catastrophizing independently predict functioning in patients with chronic pain? *Pain, 85,* 115-125.

Van Houdenhove, B. (1986). Prevalence and psychodynamic interpretation of premorbid hyperactivity in patients with chronic pain. *Psychotherapy and Psychosomatics, 45,* 195-200.

Van Middelkoop, M., Rubinstein, S. M., Ostelo, R., van Tulder, M. W., Peul, W., Koes, B. W., & Verhagen, A. P. (2012). Surgery versus conservative care for neck pain: A systematic review. *European Spine Journal, 22(1),* 87-95. doi: 10.1007/s00586-012-2553-z

Van Praag, H., Jacobs, B. L., Gage, F. H. (2000). Depression and the birth and death of brain cells. *American Scientist, 88,* 340-345.

Viane, I., Crombez, G., Eccleston, C., Poppe, C., Devulder, J., Van Houdenhove, B., & De Cote, W. (2003). Acceptance of pain is an independent predictor of mental well-being in patients with chronic pain: Empirical evidence and reappraisal. *Pain, 106,* 65-72.

Vlaeyen, J. W., & Linton, S. J. (2000). Fear-avoidance and its consequences in chronic musculoskeletal pain: A state of the art. *Pain, 85,* 317-332.

Von Korff, M., Dworkin, S. F., & La Resche, L. (1990). Graded chronic pain status: An epidemiologic evaluation. *Pain, 40,* 279-291.

Vuong. C., Van Uum, S. H., O'Dell, L. E., Lutfy, K., & Friedman, T. C. (2010). The effects of opioids and opioid analogs on animal and human endocrine systems. *Endocrine Review, 31*, 98-132.

Waddell, G., Newton, M., Henderson, I., Somerville, D., & Main, C. J. (1993). A fear-avoidance behavior questionnaire (FABQ) and the role of fear-avoidance beliefs in chronic low back pain and disability. *Pain, 52*, 157-168.

Wegener, S. T., Castillo, R. C., Haythornwaite, J., MacKenzie, E. J., & Bosse, M. J. (2011). Psychological distress mediates the effect of pain on function. *Pain, 152*, 1349-1357.

Weiner, B. K., & Levi, B. H. (2004). The profit motive and spine surgery. *Spine, 29, 22*, 2588-2591.

Wieseler-Frank, J., Maier, S. F., & Watkins, L. R. (2005). Immune-to-brain communication dynamically modulates pain: Physiological and pathological consequences. *Brain, Behavior, & Immunity, 19*, 104-111.

Williams, J. W., Mulrow, C. D., Chiquette, E., Noel, P. H., Aguilar, C., & Cornell, J. (2000). A systematic review of new pharmacotherapies for depression in adults: Evidence report summary. *Annals of Internal Medicine, 132*, 743-756.

Woolf, C. J. (2011). Central sensitization: Implications for the diagnosis and treatment of pain. *Pain, 152 (3 Suppl)*, S2-15.

Woolf, C. J., & Salter, M. W. (2000). Neuronal plasticity: Increasing the gain in pain. *Science, 288*, 1765-1768.

Yi, R., Kohno, T., Moore, K. A., & Woolf, C. J. (2003). Central sensitization and LTP: Do pain and memory share similar mechanisms? *Trends in Neuroscience, 26*, 696-705.

Yunus, M. B. (2007). The role of central sensitization in symptoms beyond muscle pain, and the evaluation of a patient with widespread pain. *Best Practice Research in Clinical Rheumatology, 21*, 481-497.

About the Author

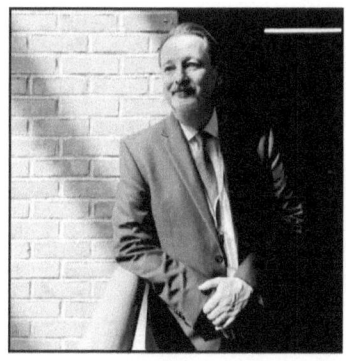

Dr. McAllister founded the Institute for Chronic Pain, an educational and public policy think tank with the mission to change the culture of how pain is managed.

He also served as Clinical Director of Pain Services for Courage Kenny Rehabilitation Institute, part of Allina Health–the fifth largest rehabilitation provider network in the United States. He held a Doctor of Psychology degree from Antioch University, New England.

Dr. McAllister passed away before this book was published, but his writing, research and ground breaking approach live on as a gift of hope to those who live with chronic pain.

www.ingramcontent.com/pod-product-compliance
Lightning Source LLC
Chambersburg PA
CBHW050854150626
46549CB00013B/1659